THE **PROSTATE CANCER** REVOLUTION

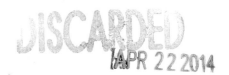

THE

PROSTATE CANCER REVOLUTION

*Beating Prostate Cancer
Without Surgery*

ROBERT L. BARD, MD

With a chapter on focal laser treatment by Dan Sperling, MD
Edited by Karen Barrie, MS

NEW YORK

THE **PROSTATE CANCER** REVOLUTION
Beating Prostate Cancer Without Surgery

© 2014 **ROBERT L. BARD, MD.**

Published in New York, New York, by Morgan James Publishing. Morgan James and The Entrepreneurial Publisher are trademarks of Morgan James, LLC.
www.MorganJamesPublishing.com

The Morgan James Speakers Group can bring authors to your live event. For more information or to book an event visit The Morgan James Speakers Group at www.TheMorganJamesSpeakersGroup.com.

DISCLAIMER: The information in this book is for educational purposes only and is not a substitute for professional medical care. Dr. Robert Bard and the Biofoundation for Angiogenesis R & D

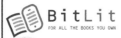

FREE eBook edition for your existing eReader with purchase

_____

PRINT NAME ABOVE

For more information, instructions, restrictions, and to register your copy, go to **www.bitlit.ca/readers/register** or use your QR Reader to scan the barcode:

ISBN 978-1-61448-905-4 paperback
ISBN 978-1-61448-906-1 eBook
ISBN 978-1-61448-908-5 hardcover
Library of Congress Control Number:
2013947438

Cover Design by:
Rachel Lopez
www.r2cdesign.com

Interior Design by:
Bonnie Bushman
bonnie@caboodlegraphics.com

In an effort to support local communities, raise awareness and funds, Morgan James Publishing donates a percentage of all book sales for the life of each book to Habitat for Humanity Peninsula and Greater Williamsburg.

Get involved today, visit
www.MorganJamesBuilds.com

Habitat
for Humanity®
Peninsula and
Greater Williamsburg
Building Partner

MEDICAL TEXTBOOKS BY DR BARD

DCE-MRI of Prostate Cancer (Springer 2009)

Image Guided Prostate Cancer Treatments (Springer 2013)

HEALTH BOOKS BY DR BARD

Prostate Cancer Decoded

Prostate Cancer Demystified

Focused Prostate Cancer Treatments

MEDICAL BOOKS CO-AUTHORED BY DR BARD

Ultrasonography of the Abdomen

Ultrasonography of the Pelvis

Ultrasonography of the Eye

Imaging of the Foot

Diagnostic Ultrasonography of Skin Cancer

DEDICATION

To my patients, whose courage showed me possiblity

To my wife, Loreto, whose vision generated results

TABLE OF CONTENTS

Foreword   *xv*

Preamble   *xvii*

Prologue   *xix*

CHAPTER 1   Taking the Risk to Change   1

CHAPTER 2   Understanding the Facts   14

CHAPTER 3   Medical Truths Are Not Sacred Cows   20

CHAPTER 4   Practical Anatomy, Pathology and Diagnosis   34

CHAPTER 5   Trust Experience and Gather Information   53

CHAPTER 6   Focal Laser Ablation of Prostate Tumors   58

CHAPTER 7   Assessing Treatment Response   71

CHAPTER 8   Reflections on Conventional Treatments   75

CHAPTER 9   Promising Scientific Breakthroughs   83

CHAPTER 10   Boosting The Body's Defenses   109

CHAPTER 11   Cancer Screening Pro's and Con's   120

CHAPTER 12   An Open Mind Is Your Best Friend   129

Epilogue   *141*

Acknowledgments   *143*

Appendices   *145*

You see things: and you say, "Why?"
But I dream things that never were: and say, "Why not?"
—George Bernard Shaw

AUTHOR'S BACKGROUND

Diplomat American Board of Radiology
Member American College of Radiology
Clinical Associate Professor of Radiology New York Medical College
Director, Bio-foundation for Angiogenesis Research and Development
Advisory Board, International Musculoskeletal Ultrasound Society
High Intensity Focused Ultrasound Certification-Prostate Cancer Imaging
Member, International Cancer Imaging Society
Member, Societe d'Imagerie Ultrasonore
Member, Societe d'Imagerie Genito-Urinaire
Member, Societe Francaises de Radiologie
Member, American Society of Lasers in Medicine and Surgery
High Frequency Ultrasound Coordinator for
American Institute of Ultrasound in Medicine

FOREWORD

By Professor David Khayat, MD, PhD
President of the International Cancer Society (Paris, France)

With an estimated 238,590 new cases in 2013, prostate cancer is the most common cancer in men in USA. One man in 6 will be diagnosed with this disease in his lifetime. It is, at the same time, the second biggest killer in men, with an estimated 29,720 deaths in 2013 in the United States.

As for other cancers in the past, the science of prostate cancer has changed tremendously during the last ten years. Pre-malignant conditions have been described leading to an extremely active search for genomic signatures of prostate cell transformation. Cohort studies are ongoing. The diagnosis of prostate cancer has become more sophisticated with the introduction of newer criteria, outside of the classical Gleason classification, that could predict an individual's tumor aggressiveness, with the hope of better and more personalized tailored therapeutic strategies.

Among them, "watchful follow-up" is more widely accepted and fewer patients are getting an unnecessary prostatectomy, that, due to the widely increased use of PSA screening that occurred during the last decade, was the reason for some real concerns, both in terms of individual risk as well as for the economy of cancer.

All the tools that constituted the classical armamentarium in the management of prostate cancer have had an impressive evolution toward high sophistication and better indication: Surgery with the unquestionable benefit of the robotic technologies. Radiotherapy with the IMRT and endo brachytherapy and ARC-Therapy. Hormonal treatment with two newly approved medicines such as Abiraterone and Enzalutamide and others in clinical developments. Chemotherapy also with Docetaxel and Cabazitaxel.

Finally, prostate cancer, which was for years a disease with very few options, and not really well understood, is now a field of great change, evolving knowledge, and the focus of ongoing basic and translational research.

There is another field of particular attention regarding prostate cancer: this is the diagnostic procedures. Anatomical imaging, functional imaging as well as molecular imaging appear today as useful tools that as an oncologist, one needs to know and understand.

Acquiring this knowledge and these skills in order to improve the management of patients is a real challenge. This is where Robert L. Bard and his colleagues have contributed tremendously, through this fantastic book, to help us in decoding what is significant prostate cancer and offering revolutionary treatments.

Each chapter of this book is a kind of Bible where all existing information in the different scopes that ultimately defines the everlasting, so rapidly evolving field of prostate cancer is explained. Rarely has so much useful data been put together with such efficient communication style as in *The Prostate Cancer Revolution*.

I already advised all my assistants to read it carefully as I am sure that it will certainly help to improve our patients' outcomes worldwide.

PREAMBLE

Nothing in life is to be feared. It is only to be understood.
Now is the time to understand more, so that we may fear less.
—Marie Curie

Finally, the doctor became the patient. My role reversal was the result of having found my own prostate tumor. I had undergone an MRI for back pain and the prostate outline seemed abnormal. I performed my own sonogram and saw a small anterior (front) tumor that an examining finger could only miss, being limited to feeling the posterior (rear) side surface of the gland. I knew from my scan that the tumor was not aggressive, but it approached the outer capsule of the gland and could possibly break out of the protective covering at some later point. I decided to put my ass on the line and in the MRI scanner again. After local anesthesia, the tumor was painlessly biopsied. The biopsy confirmed nonaggressive disease several days later. However, not knowing the biopsy results, I immediately underwent the laser ablation. I felt some warmth and then it was over. No catheter and so far, no side effects. No matter what the biopsy would show, I wanted the problem gone. Another reason to have the laser ablation that took less than an hour—start to finish—was to remove the worry about spreading tumor cells after the biopsy. The laser heat cauterizes (burns) the biopsy tract killing any cells that may have escaped during the procedure. This is why it makes sense to destroy the suspicious area at the time of biopsy before the potential cancer cells can spread into other tissues.

PROLOGUE

CHRISTMAS 2012: The white haired professor of surgery suddenly stood up in the middle of the university center medical conference, glared at the presenter and pointedly said: "How can this test be accurate? For half a century", he continued, "I could tell a patient with liver metastases from malignant melanoma just by looking at the patient. Anyone with a glass eye and a bulging liver had a certain diagnosis of metastatic uveal (eye) melanoma to the liver. And you are saying that the $5,000 PET (positron emission radiation) scan cannot reliably show this?"

Unfortunately, some of these expensive tests have limitations; many of them also involve exposure to radiation. Many of the radioactive procedures lack some degree of specificity. We have developed non-radioactive imaging technologies that are replacing many older modalities and are proving more useful for diagnosis and follow up of many diseases. Breakthroughs in computerized ultrasound and robotic MRI systems are leading the path to simpler and better diagnosis and treatment applications.

As these treatments have improved dramatically in effectiveness, education of the medical profession and the patient population must be addressed to ensure that these modalities are discussed and possibly offered. As a patient, you are welcome to show this book to your physician. If he has any questions, all the data can be found on the internet or my website, www.bardcancercenter.com. I will also be happy to speak with a physician about what is possible for his/her patient. I will not be available to discuss the fact that so few physicians have this equipment or even understand this worldwide technology.

"You will die in 6 months without immediate surgery"

John leaned back in his chair. Then he straightened up, looked his doctor in the eye and said, "I will take my chances and wait." That was seventeen years ago. John had prostate carcinoma (cancer). His physician did not tell him that only 3% of prostate cancer was lethal. Unaware of the favorable odds (97% chance that his tumor was nonaggressive), John's inner faith helped him to avoid the unfavorable and likely side effects of surgery, hormones and radiation.

John died in 2008. His well-intentioned doctor at that time didn't realize the natural history of minimally aggressive prostate cancer and had been indoctrinated by the medical profession to dismiss alternative medicine as useless, if not dangerous.

I am struck by the increasing number of patients opting for homeopathic therapies and the high percentage of survivors with tumors who see me for assistance. As a diagnostic radiologist, I am not a treating physician, yet people flock to my office looking for reassurance that their chosen treatments are working. Patients taking charge of their medical care and outcomes were unwelcome in the medical milieu of the last century.

I use my imaging technologies to show the progress of cancer treatment because I had a similar experience with the "culture" of medicine in the past. After polio at age 4, my legs started failing. The doctors at the rehabilitation center specializing in this nationwide epidemic had already warned my parents I would never walk again. Even as I felt some sensation coming back in my legs, we were told I would be crippled for life. Thirteen years after I was told I would be paralyzed, I became certified as a Red Cross Water Safety Instructor and taught lifesaving techniques to lifeguards. I was very happy to prove medical science wrong.

How did this distrust of medical diagnosis and prognosis happen?

I was in the hospital recovering from paralytic polio during the worldwide epidemic in the 1940's and became short of breath. My father, a bronze star medal recipient as a physician during World War II, came in to examine me. He heard me cough, saw my dusky color, listened to my lungs, felt my hot forehead and went over to talk to my doctors. There was arguing. My father told the physician in charge I had acute pneumonia; they told him I was dying from the paralysis of my diaphragms preventing me from breathing. My father stopped talking to them, came back and whispered to me: "See these little white pills? Take one pill before each meal. Do not tell anyone else you are taking them. I will be back tomorrow." I hid the tablets under my pillow. At mealtime I decided to follow my dad's advice and ignore the specialists taking care of me. The next morning my breathing was better. As a M.A.S.H. medic, my father had brought back with him the antibiotic *penicillin* from the Pacific theater of war. It was still not widely available in the United States in 1949 and certainly not well understood. Penicillin saved the GIs' lives during the war. This antibiotic was so powerful that the medics on the battlefield could "smell" the infections of the wounded who did not have access to this wonder drug. My father saved my life by trusting his combat-tested experience rather than the advice of the so-called "experts."

I volunteered to support my country during the Vietnam conflict. With one year of radiology specialty experience, I was sent to Thailand to support the Tactical Air Command as a Captain in the U.S. Air Force. As the only USAF radiologist within 300 kilometers of Udorn Royal Thai Air Base, I assisted in diagnoses in remote places as far-flung as Thailand, Laos, Formosa, Guam, Vietnam and Cambodia. The Air Force medical facility at our base took care of the U.S. General Staff and high ranking officers of our allied forces. This was a state-of-the-art military hospital and boasted physicians of the highest caliber recruited from all over the US according to their specialties.

I also learned that in the practice of medicine, reality did not always coincide with cookbook formulations. For example, the treatment of the Cambodian colonel whose chest x-ray revealed multiple live hand-grenades buried in his chest wall could not be found in any medical textbook. There were also many different ways to treat diseases within our nation-wide American thinking and even more options employing Oriental medicine. Remember, in China, if the Chinese emperor died, so did his physician. Exposed to varied treatment possibilities, I eagerly tried to integrate Eastern medicine concepts with proven Western medicine teachings. I soon learned that there were effective alternative ways to treat many medical problems. I also observed cultural differences connected to anatomical usage. For example, the Thai people would rest by squatting. Americans, trying to fit in with local customs, quickly developed knee joint irritations. The makeup of Asian bodies had adapted to ethnic practices (or perhaps vice versa, since evolution is intertwined with behavior and environment.). Upon completion of active duty, I returned to the United States as a major and as a man who had seen diseases and treatments not common in traditional medical studies. I was humbled by the inexplicable success of Eastern remedies not readily understood by Western standards. I am even more profoundly concerned that the technologies you will read about in this book have barely penetrated the layers of our own medical community. My references are from the years 1998 to 2013. This is 15 years of proven data that should have shifted the standard of care from blind biopsies to imaging the prostate to find the so called "index lesion" that is clinically significant. Now that we can identify the killing cancer using ultrasound and MRI, image-guided methods are able to destroy tumors with major damage to the malignant cells and minimal damage to the patient.

I am writing this book to inform patients about the leading edge of medical diagnosis and new therapeutic options using image-guided treatments. I have changed my profession from "diagnostic radiologist" who saw only films to "interventional radiologist" who examines a patient and provides therapy based on the current picture of the specific disease. Treatment may be tailored for each patient based on newer concepts in radiological imaging, advanced minimally invasive treatments and on a sensitivity to the patient's personal needs and lifestyle choices.

Life without humor, according to Oscar Wilde, is not worth living. Medicine without compassion may not be worth dispensing. It is too easy today to cure the disease and destroy the patient in the process as we have witnessed with chemotherapies. This book aims at preserving human dignity and controlling cancer at the same time. My purpose in writing this book is threefold:

- to provide practical knowledge of this disease
- to offer hope and treatment options based on scientific data, and
- to encourage realistic empowerment to deal with life's medical challenges.

Not all cancer kills. In fact, most prostate cancers are now treatable without surgery. Minimally invasive treatment for benign diseases can be done in fifteen minutes while minimally invasive definitive cancer treatments may take from one to four hours. The message here is that a person need not fear prostate cancer and the risk of life-impairing treatment side effects when new and non-invasive modalities are now being utilized to detect and treat malignant tumors quickly, painlessly, and more accurately. The multiplicity of noninvasive and minimally invasive therapies with fewer side effects offers men new health choices.

CHAPTER 1

TAKING THE RISK TO CHANGE

11 PM. Emergency Department. Metropolitan Hospital. New York City, 1973. Twenty-six year old female brought in with stab wound to the chest and increasing shortness of breath. Medical team must know if there is bleeding into the pericardium, the sac that holds the heart. I confer with the heart surgeon, leave the ED and proceed to the obstetrics department. I bring back an ultrasound machine used on a pregnant woman's abdomen for determining fetal growth and place the scanner over the heart of the bleeding patient. With clear images of the extent of the injury, the patient is rushed to the OR. The surgeon, now armed with a precise picture of the site of the hemorrhage, targets his operation. The bleeding around the heart is stopped at 1:00 AM. The patient lives.

This real life story shows that a medical technology dedicated to a single use may have other potential uses. Eye scanners were used on the breast in 1978 to perceive mammary problems. Breast scanners looked at joints and tendons in 1990. Tendon imaging devices that showed blood vessels and demonstrated actual live blood flow near a joint were adapted to imaging the prostate in the mid 90's. Scanners, showing the face of the fetus using 3-Dimensional (3-D) pictures inside the uterus fifteen years ago, were soon placed on the shoulder and knee to assess injuries. Technology that improved shoulder imaging with 3-D pictures became available for the prostate ten years ago. For a while, medical imaging was mainly limited by the lack of curiosity of the physician and the paucity of semiconductor technology to make more powerful computer chips. Medical breakthroughs are sometimes as simple as thinking outside the box. There are similarities between the resistance of medical science to embrace innovations in diagnosis and treatments, and the tendency of individual persons to resist embracing constructive new ideas and behaviors. To understand how an entire profession can be slow to welcome advances, let's first examine human nature.

The following story of the "Rat and the Cheese" illustrates a how a laboratory animal changes its habit when experience showed the behavior was no longer meaningful. A rat was put in a tunnel with a piece of cheese at the end. The rat ran down the tunnel and ate the cheese. Day after day the rat was able to wend its way down the course to find unerringly the tasty morsel. One day the cheese was removed. The rat went down the tunnel and tried to find the cheese. The next day the rat entered the tunnel and searched without success. The third day the rat went into the tunnel and came out without any cheese. At the end of the fourth day the rat refused to enter the tunnel.

The difference between rats and human beings is this: the rat quickly learned what worked and what did not work, while people often continue outmoded or futile behavior patterns despite the absence of tangible rewards. For example, if one goes into a room full of people and asks those who are 10 pounds or more overweight to raise their hands, and then asks those who know that exercise and dieting will control their weight to raise their hands—the same hands go up. Being overweight is not rewarding physically or psychologically. Those who raise their hands know better, yet that knowledge is not sufficient for them to override their self-destructive habits.

Here's another example from nature. Do you know hunters trap wild monkeys? You see, these primates are similar to humans in important ways. A banana is put into a jar with a narrow neck. The monkey reaches into the jar and grabs the banana in his closed fist. The width of the clenched hand with the banana is wider than the jar opening. As the hunter comes to catch the monkey, the animal gets frantic, but will not let go of the banana. All it has to do is give up its grip—simple, but the monkey's instinct to hang onto food interferes with its ability to risk letting go for a greater good.

Unlike the rat, people often don't listen to their own experience. Instead, like the monkey, they cling to old ways. In particular, men may avoid dealing with health issues due to denial based on fear—will the treatment be worse than the disease (impotence or incontinence)? A man's first approach to a medical problem is to wait, hoping it will go away. When the condition worsens, he waits again hoping his health won't deteriorate further or that his body's natural immune defenses will come to the rescue. Finally, when he can no longer put up with the alteration of his lifestyle, the entreaties of his concerned wife or the intolerance of his physical state, he decides to get help. FEAR stops men from being proactive in their health. Women complain about the inconvenience of mammograms, yet few miss their yearly appointments. In fact, demand is so great that in New York City the current wait time for this often uncomfortable test is up to 6 months.

What's behind the fear of seeing the doctor? Patients who delay seeking medical help fall into four risk-avoidance categories:

1. The stoic, who sees sickness as unmanly or a sign of weakness
2. The worrier, who knows too much about possible medical side effects
3. The ostrich, who is in denial
4. The victim, who gets attention from others for maintaining suffering.

Then there is the perfect patient, who overcomes his fear or anxiety and attends to potential problems early.

Fear thwarts and contradicts our natural need for survival, just as the monkey gave up the long-term survival of freedom for the short-term gratification of having a banana. Fear is a physiologic byproduct of our concerns over pain, interruption of daily routine by long waits, extensive recovery periods, and possibly, death. For countless men, the idea of seeing a doctor activates these concerns. "White collar hypertension" (high blood pressure) is a real phenomenon. Our blood pressure often rises in the doctor's office with the stress of a possible serious medical condition. Relaxing and deep breathing usually lowers the number to a safe level. Other causes of fear in the doctor's office are bad childhood experiences, claustrophobia, fear of needles, fainting at the sight of blood, low pain threshold, cold examination rooms, exposing parts of the body, etc.

No matter what kind of patient you are and no matter what your fear of the unknown, don't wait till it is too late. Today's technologies and treatments are minimally invasive, removing the threat of catastrophic side effects. Thus, taking the risk to overcome this fear is one of the safest choices you can make! Tell the physician and his staff about your anxiety and request specific arrangements. For instance, while no one objects to a prostate sonogram, many men wince at the thought of being inside the claustrophobic MRI tube for half an hour. For these concerns, we may modify the procedure to keep the head outside the tube or inject anti-anxiety medicine to reduce the stress of the procedure. Newer MRI machines can reduce the scan time in half.

Here's a perfect example of the greater risk of waiting too long to seek medical help. A colleague in good health developed heartburn and treated it with antacids for two weeks. When it got worse and the acid rose up in his throat irritating the throat and voice box producing hoarseness, he called the gastroenterologist. The GI doctor told him to fast after midnight and see him at 8 AM the next morning for an endoscopy, a scope inserted through the mouth that looks at the esophagus and stomach. He had a light dinner and started the fast earlier at 10 PM. After the anesthesia wore off from the procedure, he was told the test couldn't be performed because the stomach had not emptied and the retained food contents blocked the view of the endoscope. He knew in a flash that common causes for an obstruction preventing emptying of the stomach were either a severe duodenal ulcer or cancer of the outlet end of the stomach. Since he had no real pain, he was sure he had a malignancy. He consulted me and we arrived at the understanding that worst possible outcome, cancer, might still be in an early stage. The test was repeated after a 12 hour fast and a small benign ulcer of the stomach wall was discovered which resolved in a month under routine treatment. The moral is: it is better to deal with your worst nightmare promptly than to procrastinate and lose the opportunity for a relatively painless curative treatment. The ancient philosopher, Seneca, said *"pars sanitatis velle sanari fuit"* or "the wish to be cured is part of the cure."

Now let's look at how the field of medicine often resists innovation, just as individuals are prone to do. After all, physicians are human, too. While we try to do the best for our patients, doctors are slow to let go of customary ideas and even slower to accept new concepts. Medical practitioners rightfully demand proof that a change from a tried and true routine will make sense before adopting a new method, but how much proof is "enough"? My former partner and late colleague, Dr. Selig Strax, Professor of Surgery at Mount Sinai Medical Center in New York, also commented on the tendency of the medical profession's avoidance of change. Half a century ago, he introduced the first "lumpectomy" operation (to remove a malignant tumor while conserving the breast) at Mount Sinai. It took a quarter century longer for this proven method to be uniformly adopted throughout the national medical community. The original radical mastectomy surgical operation, removing the entire breast, chest wall muscles, and occasionally part of the rib cage, was based on the 100-year old idea that cancer spreads in linear progression to nearby tissues. After the discovery that small cancers could infiltrate the lymph nodes (glands) and from there spread widely to every other organ through the blood stream, did the radical mastectomy cease? No. For the next thirty years this mutilating procedure was the gold standard of breast cancer therapy in spite of growing proof that it had outlived its purpose. Breast surgeons clung to their traditional methods, nor was there much demand from patients. Why? Before the Information Age when computers and the internet became commonplace, women didn't have easy access to accurate and understandable information about the lumpectomy procedure. Today's prostate cancer patient, on the other hand, is armed with the internet, the news media and national prostate cancer support groups and programs. Men need not acquiesce to their doctors who recommend one specific treatment or dictate their own preferred therapy. The information revolution allows men to research and choose the best available medical options for their particular condition and level of comfort with the stated potential risks. Think about how you would like your life after prostate cancer to be. As Einstein once put it, "Imagination is more important than knowledge"

If I propose the "prostate lumpectomy," how long will it take the scientific community to consider the possibility? This book proposes simple, straightforward and logical alternatives to currently accepted "gold standard" conventional treatments. Many of these advanced alternative diagnostic modalities and therapeutic procedures are now common practice in Europe, Asia, South America and other civilized countries around the globe.

Making the leap: clinical trial and anecdotal observation

There are two important phrases in classic scientific methodology: clinical trial and anecdotal observation. Clinical trial is evidence accumulated based on an assumption of a possible mechanism of therapy to be investigated. Anecdotal observation means that a treatment worked once or twice, and the mechanism may not be readily understood at that time. The *bard* of modern times says, "To succeed, or not to succeed—that is the question." **It is more useful to have a treatment that works and is not understood than to have a therapy that makes sense but ultimately fails**. A beef steak placed over a black eye helps, but the cold and pressure of an ice pack would do better to reduce the pain and swelling. Likewise, dabbing tincture of iodine over a cut will sterilize the wound yet produce more tissue damage due to its high local tissue toxicity. The following example shows how the interplay between formal clinical study and anecdotal evidence can drive medicine forward.

The drug *finasteride* (Proscar®) was developed fifteen years ago as a miracle cure for progressive urinary symptoms of an enlarged prostate. Initial clinical trials showed it was useful and Proscar rapidly received FDA approval. Early studies also suggested that it might reduce prostate cancer risk. Anecdotal reports that it was only minimally effective began to appear and increase in number. New data also suggested men were developing serious cancers while on the medication. Finally, a critique of a large study recently concluded, surprisingly, that while the drug was somewhat useful in alleviating the symptoms of benign prostatic hypertrophy, and there was an overall 25% decrease in prostate cancer prevalence, there was a 68% increase in the frequency of high grade killing prostate cancers in the treated group. This report, published in the 2004 *Journal of Urology* by Dr. Patrick Walsh (Johns Hopkins Medical Center) underscores the interaction between clinical trials and anecdotal reports. A study from the National Cancer Institute on this subject was presented by Dr. Lucia in the 2005 issue of *The Journal of Urology*. It indicated that the high grade cancers (Gleason 8-10) induced by *finasteride* were limited to one side rather than both sides of the prostate gland thus validating Dr. Walsh's findings. The wonder drug appeared to produce fewer nonlethal tumors but stimulate more aggressive killing cancers. Clearly more research must focus on the controversial area of cancers being aggravated by prescription medications.

The story does not end here. Since the evidence didn't fit the theory, the facts were reinterpreted in the last few years. It is now felt that the increase in significant tumors was due to the shrinking of the enlarged prostate that made the more dangerous cancer easier to detect. The jury is still out in this trial and we need more data to come to a definitive conclusion. A major study on breast cancer demonstrated 10% of proven cancers disappeared after six years without treatment. Remember, the breast and prostate are both glands. Like breast cancers, we see some prostate cancers resolve without traditional medical treatments and this possibility deserves further clinical study.

David Hess in the Rutgers University Press publication (1999), *Evaluating Alternative Cancer Therapies*, quotes the following from medical scholar Robert Houson:

> The FDA requires a convincing mechanism to obtain approval for clinical trials, and I think this is a completely unnecessary requirement. If there are clear indications of benefit in humans or animals, that should bypass the whole issue of mechanism. The point is that the investigators do not have to know the mechanism in order to corroborate the effect that is occurring. In cancer, case studies have a greater degree of validity than in other diseases. In cancer the rate of spontaneous remission is extremely low, so low that it is virtually zero. Therefore, if you have just a few cases, even only two cases, you have something that is significant and most likely meaningful. So, I consider what is being dismissed as anecdotal evidence, to be in cancer, actually an impressive proof of success because you can have much more detail in the case studies than you can in a clinical trial.

The same principle of anecdotal observation applies to advances in disease detection through imaging. In the 1980's, when the state of the art sonogram equipment showed that doctors could see malignant lymph nodes (cancerous glands), I started a protocol with Cabrini Medical Center in New York City under the famed breast surgeon, Dr. Henry Leis. We scanned patients with breast cancer to see if the underarm lymph nodes were involved by tumor. Detection of these cancerous glands meant surgery was not indicated, since abnormal glands showed the cancer had spread too far for a local operation to be useful. The results of our investigation spared selected patients unnecessary surgery. The project broke new ground and showed that the sonogram accurately detected larger cancerous glands, thereby saving some patients from the operating room. We also discovered certain types of highly aggressive breast cancers seemed to shrink the breast instead of producing a lump. In these patients, the mammogram was read as "normal" even though the contracted breast tissue was hard as a rock at the physical examination. This variety of cancer produced scarring and retraction of the tissues as it grew. The mammogram was useless in the diagnosis, but because we were willing to "risk" applying a different technology we learned that the sonogram visualized them easily. Our leap of faith paid off. The hospital began a screening program for high-risk patients which in turn led to the discovery of malignancies at very early stages. This has increased the amount of surgery and decreased the spread of cancer, resulting in more favorable outcomes.

The experimental use of ultrasound technology led to an investigational clinical trial after anecdotal cases pointed the way to a specific treatment protocol. The same lymph node sonography is currently being used in Europe to determine the possible spread of other cancers, especially the deadly skin tumor malignant melanoma. If the major lymph nodes draining the tumorous area are unremarkable, extensive disfiguring biopsy may now be avoided. If an abnormal lymph node is found, it may be needle biopsied in a few minutes, with the cells immediately analyzed by a cytopathologist. This real time biopsy/analysis may render unnecessary a complicated combination of radiation with surgical biopsy to better stage the spread of disease throughout the lymph node chain.

My high school chemistry teacher in 1958 was Mr. Marantz. As an eager student, I had looked up some information in a journal and proudly told him I had done some "research" on a topic. He looked at me sternly, saying, "Research is not finding something in a book. Research is being committed to a project and observing and analyzing what happens during the investigation." He then related his story of how he became a school teacher. He was a topnotch industrial research chemist before he entered a teaching career. The New Jersey pharmaceutical plant he worked in was located alongside a river. Three of the walls of the laboratory were steel and concrete. The fourth wall, facing the river, was made of plasterboard and wood. He invented new substances by taking risks and boldly trying unexplored chemical pathways. From time to time there would be a fire or an explosion. On three separate occasions, the false wall, the experiment, and Mr. Marantz landed in the river. After the fourth time, he left for the (at the time) safer task of teaching high school students—but not before that last explosion resulted in the unfortunate loss of three fingers.

I, too, took a risk in forging my path in medicine. After I returned from military service in South East Asia to my radiology residency at the New York Medical College, I requested a leave from the program to attend the renowned Armed Forces Institute of Pathology (AFIP). The AFIP is the national medical teaching center specializing in correlating radiologic findings with unusual pathologic specimens throughout the U.S. and from military bases around the world. The chief of my residency allowed me three months unpaid leave to study in Washington, D.C. I remember vividly in 1973 the director of the radiology training program showing a difficult case of gonococcus urethritis (venereal disease of the male urethra) at the afternoon teaching conference. My AFIP experience of reviewing selected cases referred in from the military's worldwide theaters of operation had given me an advantage in interpreting x-rays. Thus I was the only resident in that teaching conference making the correct diagnosis. In disbelief, the director commented aloud that I must have seen the x-ray films beforehand in the urology clinic of the hospital!

By the time my third year residency was finishing, I was passionately convinced that the future of imaging lay in the new field of diagnostic ultrasound (clinical MRI was not yet invented and CT scans were in their infancy). It was the custom of the department head to sit with the residents and guide them to their future. The chief completely dismissed my enthusiasm as "impractical." Nonetheless, I took a risk, just like my chemistry teacher. This time the experiment didn't blow up. I am fortunate that the sonogram has become the primary imaging diagnostic test in international use today. As of this date, many new, previously unthinkable uses are becoming available to the medical community in this rapidly growing diagnostic field that has re-entered the treatment arena by its ability to image-guide therapies. An example is the portable hand held unit that can be carried to the patients' bedside or brought onto a football field to check for a tendon tear or a bone fracture after an injury. If an athlete has ruptured a muscle with a huge blood leak, the physician can introduce a needle under sonographic guidance and remove the blood clot. This would shorten the period of disability to days instead of months. Simply said, if a disease or tumor can be imaged by any radiologic procedure, it may be treated under direct visual observation at the same time.

There is a role for both clinical study and anecdotal evidence. Ideally, they serve the same end: medical advancement. Much of the work I am presenting is both a clinical trial and anecdotal evidence simultaneously studied and accumulated over a nineteen-year period. During this time the subject has been exhaustively evaluated and continues to evolve in design and power as newer, better and different technologies and treatments became available. I saw alternative cancer treatments work in patients. These cancer survivors came in for follow up exams, continuously, every six months to monitor their health. All the men had refused traditional medical therapies and standard surgical regimens. In short order, the mechanism of action of tumor growth revealed itself to me. Also, the possibility to use ultrasound technology for diagnostic evaluation and prognostic information predicting the longevity of the patient became obvious.

The *Rat and the Cheese* analogy helps us understand the snail-paced change in the practice of medicine. When Dr. Bertrand Guillonneau introduced the laparoscopic radical prostatectomy (LRP) procedure in Paris in 1995, he was considered radical for wanting to alter the existing established treatment. His student, Dr. Arnon Krongrad, brought this laser surgical technique to the United States in 1999, and was initially outcast by the local medical community. Later, the LRP was superseded by the robotic-assisted radical prostatectomy (RRP) but debate continued as to whether a surgeon's own hands in a patient's body would or would not be more sensitive than robotically manipulated instruments guided by extreme visual magnification. When a traditional method offers fewer rewards than an innovation does, is it not time to start questioning the norm? Acceptance of new ideas occurs slowly, and its transformation into action as distinct new protocols is frequently glacial. The information presented in this book is not new, is not hidden and is not controversial. The majority of concepts in this book have been in use internationally for over thirty years. The same way that the radical mastectomy was phased out by the breast lumpectomy, so may the traditional radical prostatectomy pass into history as a treatment that no longer serves the good of most patients. Already the standard surgical treatment for improving urine flow in men with enlarged prostates (the Trans-Urethral Resection of the Prostate or TURP) is becoming less popular among younger urologists in training programs. Indeed, the green light laser accomplishes the same effect with less blood loss and is done as an outpatient procedure. Alternatively, oral medications that relax the urinary sphincter muscle have reduced the need for any surgery by 60% in men with obstructive symptoms from an enlarged gland.

Change doesn't just come from doctors. Our patients also play a key part in propelling progress in medical practice. Patients who could drive home a few days after surgery helped increase the demand for this growing new standard of care. Less invasive prostatectomy, with its speedy recovery and lower side effect profile, is a positive trend for patients. But it's essential to ask ourselves: how many patients even require surgical prostate removal? Today's patients are not passive. Educated patients want what ***does*** work rather than what ***should*** work. Educated men are asking their doctors hard questions, yet they are not prepared to address them to their patients' satisfaction.

There is further concern surrounding current acceptable diagnostic and treatment practices, not the least of which is the reliability of the now embattled prostate specific antigen (PSA) blood test and the time honored digital rectal exam

(DRE). It is time to take the risk and rethink long-standing, traditional approaches to prostate cancer detection and the efficacy of currently accepted cures. Thus, the American Society of Preventive Medicine no longer recommends screening for prostate cancer with either the PSA or the DRE in its 2008 official policy recommendations.

Dualistic vs. integrative thinking

When we come face to face with a problem, it's tempting to oversimplify the solution as "either this or that." The name for this type of thinking is *false dichotomy*, meaning there are many more ways to resolve the situation but we've reduced ourselves to only two. Prostate cancer patients are all too familiar with the side effect risks that accompany conventional whole-gland treatments. Unless they are aware of a broad spectrum of choices, their options are limited to only two: Either it's CONVENTIONAL TREATMENT, or it's NO TREATMENT.

Thankfully, there is an entire array of therapeutic choices in the world of Complementary and Alternative Medicine (CAM). Complementary and alternative medical techniques are often seen as a middle ground between no treatment and standard conventional medicine. Perhaps each of these three options has something to recommend it. The 2008 *Archives Of Internal Medicine* featured a large study of breast cancer patients in which some of the tumors disappeared spontaneously after being observed over a six year period. Dr. Robert Kaplan from UCLA and Dr. Franz Porzsolt from the University Cancer Center in Ulm, Germany analyzed the data and suggested a reevaluation of breast cancer research and treatment be considered. Proven cancers had regressed after no treatment.

The National Institutes of Health (NIH) define conventional medicine as medicine practiced by licensed health care professionals to treat diseases using drugs, radiation or surgery. This is also termed Western, modern, mainstream or orthodox medicine. Professional schools that train students in conventional medicine award degrees that include MD (Doctor of Medicine) and DO (Doctor of Osteopathy) as well as degrees in nursing, pharmacy and practical therapies. In contrast, the NIH loosely defines CAM as a group of diverse health care systems, practices and products that are not presently considered to be part of conventional medicine. CAM practices include:

- Mind Body Medicine such as meditation, prayer, imaging and art therapy to enhance the mind's capacity to alter bodily function

- Biologically Based Practices like herbs, botanicals and dietary supplements found in nature but not yet scientifically proven to be efficacious
- Manipulative Practices including massage and chiropractic employing manipulation of the spine and other body parts
- Energy Medicine which is divided into Biofield Therapies as Qi Gong, Reiki and Acupuncture that manipulate the body to affect the "energy fields" and Bioelectromagnetic Therapies like Magnetic Therapy, Sound Energy Therapy and Light Therapy that use electromagnetic fields to produce health benefits.

In practice, CAM is categorized into complimentary medicine which is used *alongside* Western medicine, and alternative medicine which is used *in place of* potentially harmful conventional medicine. History has shown that numerous CAM therapies over time have become conventional, such as the cinchona Peruvian bark, which was the only effective treatment for malaria for more than 300 years.

The NIH created the National Center for Complimentary and Alternative Medicine (NCCAM) in 1998 to evaluate scientifically CAM therapies and transport effective treatments from CAM to traditional medicine. The organization is developing guidelines to regulate the purity and consistency of dietary supplements. Many products have different concentrations, varied packaging that affects dissolution or absorption and even poisonous lead contaminants such as found in Chinese products.

Perhaps taking the risk to change isn't as risky as it seems. The contributions of CAM are centuries-old. While much of the evidence from other cultures is anecdotal, clinical studies continue to verify the benefits of CAM modalities—in some cases, to improve upon them. In dealing with prostate cancer, physicians and patients must never fall into false dichotomies (either/or) as together we strive for treatments that ***work***, rather than continue to apply outdated treatments that are ***supposed to*** work. In the change process, we can move beyond

CONVENTIONAL VS. NO TREATMENT (false dichotomy)

and enlarge our categories into a spectrum that allows fluid movement among all categories from one end of the spectrum to the other. It would look like this:

From CAM through all treatment categories including **NO TREATMENT**

In fact, we are well on our way—as this book demonstrates—in spite of conventional medicine occasionally clinging to the banana in its clenched hand.

CHAPTER 2

UNDERSTANDING THE FACTS

A century ago, physicians were taught that cancers started with a few cells that divided, gradually enlarging to become major clusters of actively growing cells called tumors. At a certain size, the tumor would become more aggressive and begin invading adjacent organs and structures, spreading out like the tentacles of an octopus. The concept of blood borne distant spread of a local tumor appeared years later. Neither theory could account for the fact that some breast and prostate cancers would appear and remain stable over periods of up to thirty-five years without growing or metastasizing. Fifty years ago the colon polyp (small benign growth) was thought to be innocent, until it was learned that certain polyps left untreated eventually turned malignant. It's tempting to view our current reality as black or white—but there appear to be many shades of gray. Ideas of cancer generation have continually changed over time.

Sometimes physicians accept evidence that does not fully consider the totality of facts at hand, or perhaps they are not cognizant of the overall spectrum of clinical data. I acknowledge generalization is useful and necessarily makes learning easier, but diseases, and patients individually, do not conform to generalities. Let us look at "facts" currently made available to physicians and the public by the media and cancer organizations.

According to *American Cancer Society Facts and Figures 2012*, over 240,000 cases of prostate cancer are expected to be diagnosed in a single year. An estimated 28,170 men will die of this disease. Findings reported by the Centers for Disease Control and Prevention and the National Cancer Institute in collaboration with the North American Association of Central Cancer Registries show the leading type of cancer causing death among men is lung cancer; however, prostate cancer is the most common form of cancer diagnosed in men in the US.

Prostate cancer facts:

- One in 6 men will get prostate cancer.
- A man is 33% more likely to develop prostate cancer than a woman is to develop breast cancer.
- As baby boomer men reach the target zone for prostate cancer, beginning at age 50, the number of new cases is projected to increase dramatically.
- By 2015, there will be more than 300,000 new prostate cancer cases each year, an increase of one third.
- There has been no change in the US cancer death rate between 1950 and 2001.
- In this same time period, there have been decreases in the death rate for other diseases:
    Pneumonia decreased 54%
    Strokes decreased 68%
    Heart disease decreased 58%

The lifetime probability of a man in the US developing cancer is 50%. A breakdown of this data shows the lifetime cancer probability for:

1. Prostate 17%
2. Lung 8%
3. Colon 6%
4. Bladder 6%
5. Lymphoma 2%
6. Melanoma 4%
7. Leukemia 2%

8. Mouth 1%
9. Kidney 1%
10. Stomach 1%

Of this list, prostate cancer is the most common and most rapidly increasing cancer. Without improvements in diagnosis and treatment:

1. In 2015 the number of new prostate cancer cases will increase by a third
2. In 2037 there will be over 400,000 new prostate cancer cases per year
3. In 2020, the number of prostate cancer deaths per year will increase 44%
4. In 2030, 80,000 men will lose their lives to prostate cancer
(Statistical Source: Prostate Cancer Foundation 2010)

The March 2004 *News of New York* (Medical Society of the State of New York) reported:

While the latest report from the National Cancer Institute (NCI) suggests that death rates for the top cancer killers in men and women are dropping, the lifetime rate of probability of developing cancer remains at 1 in 2 for men and 1 in 3 for women.

To increase the cancer detection rate, a lowering of the threshold for biopsy is recommended. The traditional standard maintained that a level of PSA greater than 4 (normal 0-4 ng/ml) was suspicious. Some physicians are now saying this is too high and recommend that a biopsy be performed when the PSA level is above 2.5. Their reasoning is supported by journalism like the May 27, 2004 issue of the *New York Times*, which ran a piece reporting that even when the PSA is normal, "prostate cells may prove to be cancerous."

A forum on prostate cancer biopsies at the 2004 International Congress of Radiology found that the PSA often rises following a biopsy, which then leads to another biopsy to determine the reason for the elevated PSA, which would in turn further raise the PSA resulting in another biopsy to rule out cancer based on a rising PSA level. One patient was given a series of five biopsies of six needles each (totaling 30 punctures) over four years due to rising PSA levels. Cancer was never found. No physician on the panel of experts made the connection that the trauma of the biopsy procedure by itself, not a cancer, may have generated higher PSA levels. A variety of causes have been demonstrated to elevate PSA levels, including tumor, trauma, inflammation and benign hypertrophy. Dr. Hattangadi et al in the December, 2012 *British Journal of Urology* (Vol 110 Issue 11) noted that in men with a PSA below 2.5, the digital rectal exam (DRE) was accurate in detecting high grade prostate cancer tumors (Gleason 8, 9. 10). A similar study seven years earlier, presented by Dr. J. Slaton at the 100th American Urological Association (AUA) Annual Meeting (2005) noted that the DRE was more accurate in detecting high grade cancers than the PSA. In a series of 3817 patients, it was determined that the most highly aggressive tumors generated low amounts of PSA. While only 685 (0.4%) of the 166,104 men in the Hattangadi study actually fell into this category, their chances of survival improved because such tumors were treatable. In other words, PSA alone is not necessarily indicative of whether prostate cancer exists or not in any given man. The same issue contained an article by Drs. Boniol and Boyle et al acknowledged that the efficacy of PSA screening was debatable, with random studies revealing inconclusive data. In fact, "even using the hypothesis most favorable to prostate cancer screening with PSA, the net number of years of life does not favour screening." To go a step further, their study demonstrated that biopsies resulting from PSA screening actually decreased survival by 3.6 years of life per avoided death. In particular, they critically examined the Swedish arm of a large-scale body of European screening data. They found that in Sweden the biopsy rate is 40% whereas in Europe it is 27%. The Swedish treatment rate was 4.1% as opposed to the 3.4% European rate, and the result of the overtreatment generated more harm than good.

Questions, questions everywhere...

What do these facts mean? Is there really an epidemic? Should men over 45 get biopsies? Do men over 40 need yearly PSA blood tests? These questions will be answered in the following pages, but two questions remains that can be answered now:

1. Is there a way to avoid biopsies? The answer to that question is a resounding YES and comes from the international pioneer in prostate cancer imaging, Dr. Francois Cornud, Professor of Interventional Radiology at Necker University Hospital in France. In 1990 Dr. Cornud began using a new technology in Paris called color Doppler ultrasound which showed abnormal blood vessels in aggressive prostate cancers. His first textbook

on this subject was published in French during 1993. A 2005 version by Dr. Olivier Helenon contains 1,424 pages of medical text using the latest diagnostic imaging methodologies. Textbooks by Dr. Cornud and Dr. Roy both appeared in 2006 and 2011 on the updated version of the same topics. A French oncologist, Dr. C. Cuenod, commented at the 2012 International European Radiology Convention; "le degree de la neoangiogenese est correlee a l'agressivite tumorale au risque de metastases" which means, the more vascular a tumor or the more blood vessels within it, the greater the risk of spread. This idea was repeated at the 2012 Journees Francaises de Radiologie with presentations by me and by investigators at the French Cancer Institute noting that 3D blood flow imaging correlates best with aggressive cancer diagnosis. Recent conferences worldwide are now recommending a tumor of low grade up to 14 (fourteen) mm in diameter may be safely followed using such imaging. This has been updated from the 8 mm diameter previous recommendation.

2. Is there a better way do biopsies? Again the answer is YES. The current accuracy of sonography and MRI now allows us to target the killing or dominant tumor.[1] Many prostate tumors of low danger are scattered throughout the gland and are suitable for observation at yearly intervals. The serious cancers are generally well imaged by the newer Doppler flow sonograms and 3T MRI units. Indeed, a useful MRI grading system has been established to assess the seriousness of the abnormal finding with a score from 0-15. Clearly a number closer to 15 requires a targeted biopsy as contrasted to a much lower number such as 3 or 4. Using Doppler computer analysis, similarly, a tumor with low vessel density of 1-4 is probably low grade while a focus with tumor vessel density greater than 10 is most likely a dangerous lesion.

A review of the facts, then, suggests that the incidence of prostate cancer is likely to increase over the coming years. However, the PSA blood test can give just so much information. Likewise, the DRE can be useful in detecting high grade

---

1   "Many prostate cancers when you analyze a radical prostatectomy (RP) specimen, have several separate tumor nodules. In most of these cases, there is one major tumor nodule which has the highest Gleason score and is the most aggressive and is called the dominant or index tumor nodule. There may be smaller lower grade cancers elsewhere in the prostate which adds no prognostic significance. A new concept is focal therapy for prostate cancer..."
(Source: www.talkabouthealth.com/dominant-tumor)

tumors that are not suggested by a low PSA value. Moreover, the rush to biopsy using traditional "blind" methods may do more harm than good.

With this in mind, the important chapters ahead cover new sonogram and MRI technologies that alter the fundamental nature of cancer diagnosis and offer elegant and rational advanced treatment options with fewer side effects.

CHAPTER 3

MEDICAL TRUTHS ARE NOT SACRED COWS

"Una sola esperienza o concludente dimonstrazione…basta a battere in terra questi ed altri centomila argomenti probabili" ("A single experience or conclusive demonstration is enough to defeat 100,000 possible arguments.")
—**Galileo Galilei**, 16th century

"Open your textbook to page 89 and *tear it out*," said my Professor of Medicine in 1965. I could hardly believe my ears! However, I and the entire second year class of '68 at the Upstate Medical Center of the State University of New York obediently opened up our brand new pathology texts and tore out the page on inflammation as he declared, "Medical knowledge is not perfect and knowledge is not a substitute for wisdom or experience." His words echoed in the lecture hall. "After all, bloodletting was the medical standard for hundreds of years," he continued. My first awareness that medicine is art as well as science was born in that moment.

In 1986, I saw a young Irish woman and did a sonogram on her abdomen. This was unremarkable, and I asked her again why she was being examined. "Don't you remember me from two years ago? Don't you recall I was told I had three months to live back then?" she replied. I looked up her old chart and found pictures showing that she had widespread breast cancer that had metastasized to the liver, bones and abdominal glands at that time consistent with death within three to six months. "What did you do?" I asked. She answered, "I took vitamin C and prayed." I repeated my ultrasound study confirming total absence of abdominal disease and realized that alternative treatments had a potential role in modern medicine. Perhaps there was an art to various complementary therapies as well?

A similar awakening occurred in 1995 at a breast cancer conference hosted by New York University School of Medicine. The morning lecture by the famous Swedish mammography expert Dr. Lazlo Tabar showed that a breast cancer measuring under 10 mm (1/3 inch) in size had a 99% cure rate in five years by simply removing the tumor (localized surgical lumpectomy). That afternoon, a chemotherapist of equal medical stature told the audience that chemotherapy and radiation treatments were routinely given for this type of cancer after surgical removal. The Swedish doctor jumped up and cried: "Didn't you hear my statistics this morning? What are you saying? No! What are you doing?"

I had a special reason for attending that conference. A dear friend had just been diagnosed with low grade breast cancer and asked me to search out new possibilities. Breast and prostate cancers have many clinical similarities since both are glands, and new breast cancer therapies may influence the development of new prostate cancer treatments. As I heard the different opinions of the lecturers, I was concerned with the wide variety of "standards." For example, my friend had a frozen biopsy (immediate pathologic report) on her cancer at a university hospital in New York. In order to obtain optimum results, surgeons at Harvard wait three days for the specimen to be thoroughly prepared before looking at the biopsy material under a microscope. After leaving the conference, I advised her that watching this slow growing cancer was a distinct possibility as well. She had her mastectomy the very next day. The fear of a potential negative prognosis (unfavorable predicted outcome) had crippled her ability to consider any reasonable alternative health options.

Questioning heart attack causes

Ten years ago physicians began questioning the value of bypass surgery for coronary artery disease. This led to more vigorous investigation of the mechanism of heart attacks. Dr. Eric Topol, an Interventional Cardiologist at the Cleveland Clinic, called into question the unchallenged idea that narrowing of the coronary arteries causes heart attacks. The prevailing assumption of cardiology worldwide has been that fixing a narrowed artery to the heart will help the patient's heart do better. Traditional medicine has held the idea that coronary artery disease is akin to sludge building up in a pipe. Plaque (sludge) builds up over years along blood vessel walls and eventually clogs the artery causing a heart attack by blocking the blood supply to the heart. It was believed bypass surgery or angioplasty (using balloons to push back plaque in the arteries) would open the narrowed arteries and keep them from closing up completely. It was assumed this surgical intervention would prevent heart attacks.

Research from centers around the world has brought a new concept to light. The old idea that heart attacks occur from arteries narrowed by plaque is no longer the predominant model for therapy. The dangerous plaque is soft, fragile and produces no symptoms. However, in up to 80% of cases the plaque itself is not the source of blockage. Rather, heart attacks occur when an area of plaque inside the vessel wall bursts, causing a clot to develop over this region. It is the enlarging blood clot that blocks the artery. This region of diseased artery would not be seen by electrocardiograms, angiograms, stress tests or echocardiograms. However, thanks to persistent review of previously unquestioned assumptions, better imaging technologies can identify the vulnerable area. New intra-arterial sonogram systems presented at the 2012 International Society of Endovascular Therapy Meeting are now detecting these life threatening regions.

This finding explains the fact that most heart attacks occur at 4:00 a.m. when people are sleeping and not stressed. It explains the fact that most coronaries happen unexpectedly, without the warning of chest pain. For example, a jogger, the very picture of health, may run three miles effortlessly on one day and die of a heart attack the next. If a narrowed artery was the culprit, then the exercise of running would have produced angina (severe cardiac pain). Heart patients tend to have hundreds of vulnerable plaques. The rationale of unplugging one or two arteries no longer makes sense. Researchers are also finding that plaque and heart attack risk can change dramatically and quickly. Dr. Peter Libby of Harvard Medical School recently said, "The disease is more mutable than we thought."

There has been much study on the role of inflammation producing the bursting of the arterial plaque. Pathologists now report that inflammation in the arterial wall with plaque is now a common observation and probable cause for fatal myocardial infarcts (heart attacks). Thus, the pivotal role of aspirin in preventing heart attacks may be as much due to its anti-inflammatory properties as well as the proven anticlotting mechanism.

Years ago my father, a still vigorous man and newly retired physician, was given only six months to live. At age 80 he developed mild abdominal pains after eating. His electrocardiogram was slightly abnormal. After he had his cardiac catheterization (dye study of the coronary heart arteries) he expected to be dismissed the next day. No one came to see him until a full two days after the procedure. The hospital cardiologists had reviewed it with several teams of doctors and finally told him that all his arteries were narrowed so badly that they had nothing to offer him other than the advice to get his affairs in order. I remember standing at his bedside, saying, "We'll find some way to help you, Dad," though at the time I had no idea what it would be. I sent word of my father's problem to friends in and out of the medical community. A week later, a friend brought me an article from the *New York Times* by Dr. Dean Ornish revealing a vegetarian diet could reverse atherosclerosis (thickening of the artery wall due to plaque buildup). My father went on a strict diet and his coronary symptoms gradually subsided.

At age 87, my father developed cancer of the bile ducts, a very slow growing form of tumor. Due to his diagnostic history of end stage heart disease, curative surgery was not proposed, and he had stents (tubes) inserted into the bile duct to keep the tumor from blocking the flow of bile from the gallbladder to the digestive tract. Since he did not have definitive surgical removal of the very small initial tumor, the growth kept intermittently blocking the bile flow through the tubing. He would return to the hospital every three months to have the bile duct reopened. Gradually, he became depressed, as do so many patients with chronic diseases and the quality of life alterations that accompany endlessly ongoing treatments. One Sunday morning my mother called me saying, "Come quickly. I think your father is dying. He can't get out of bed." I rushed over to see him and found him barely responsive to my questions. Finally, I shouted, "Get up! We are going for Sunday brunch at the country club. Put on your clothes." With a great deal of coaxing he dressed, got into the car and drove with us to the club. A small hill stretched between us from the parking lot to the dining room. "Dad," I said, "hold my arm and we'll walk up the hill together." He took one step, hesitated, then took another, hesitated again, and yet another. Halfway up this painstaking climb, he stopped. Smiling as he paused and looked at me, he said, "You don't have to help me now. I can walk the rest of the way by myself." And he did. Six and a half years after he was supposed to succumb to his heart disease, he had beaten the odds and reversed most of the coronary arterial plaque. When he ultimately died from his cancer, he was no longer on heart medication. As a traditionally trained physician practicing radiology, I did not fully believe in miracles until one occurred within my own family. The assumption that medical "truths" are sacred cows thus got another nail in the coffin.

While new ideas are not quickly recognized and change is often resisted, that short journey from my father's "grave" to the country club was a very big step for me. I saw how old notions tend to persist in today's medicine. The difficulties in bringing oncology innovations and unorthodox treatments to the medical marketplace may require courage. People who said the earth revolves around the sun were burned as heretics 600 years ago. While we no longer submit innovators to such dire treatment, the inherent resistance to progress serves as a template of potential pressures against developing and disseminating new concepts in cancer diagnosis and treatment. What would happen to the American Cancer Society if cancer was finally cured?

Rethinking fundamental concepts

The understanding of heart attack prevention changed only after years of research that initially met disbelief. In 1986, Dr. Greg Brown of the University of Washington in Seattle published a paper showing heart attacks occurred in areas of coronary arteries where there was too little plaque to use a stent or to use bypass surgery. He was derided by many cardiologists. Around that time Dr. Steven Nissen of the Cleveland Clinic started looking at patient's coronary arteries with a tiny ultrasound camera and proposed the idea that the "hard" plaque that obstructed arteries was not the plaque that caused heart attack. It was the "soft" plaque that was grew quickly and burst that eventually produced the fatal coronary thrombosis. He too was greeted with skepticism by his peers. In 1999, Dr. Waters from University of California received a similar reaction to his study of patients without chest pain referred for angioplasty. He found that patients who went on a cholesterol lowering diets had fewer heart attacks than those who had angioplasty (catheter opening of the arteries). Even worse was the finding by Dr. Topol who discovered that the procedure of placing a stent (tube that mechanically opens a narrowed area) in a patient's diseased arteries can actually cause minor heart attacks in about 4% of patients. This adds up to unacceptable risk of heart damage to people who chose a treatment to prevent it.

Why some cancer therapies fail

In 2004 a front-page article in the *Wall Street Journal* reported on why certain cancer therapies utilizing standard medical principles don't work as well as expected. According to the report, there are resistant stem cells that create invasiveness in cancers. These cells will keep dividing and growing while other less hardy cancer cells die off after a few growth periods. This may explain the phenomenon of cancers regressing under radiotherapy, chemotherapy or hormonal therapy only to return as more aggressive cancers later. Such recurrence was common in men treated with the Chinese herb mixture that was marketed under the name PC-SPES (P=prostate, C=cancer and "spes" is the Latin word for HOPE). This nontraditional Oriental blend shrunk the prostate, reduced an elevated PSA test to negligible values and stopped not only the cancer but many times arrested growth of the metastatic disease as well. The existence of resistant cancer stem cells also explains tumor recurrence after surgery where the margins are considered clean. In various medical series it has been shown that tumor cells may be hiding in the postoperative site. Indeed, work by Dr. Fred Lee, inventor of the ultrasound guided prostate biopsy, showed by specialized diagnostic imaging scans that about half of the clinically localized cancers have actually spread outside the prostate at surgery.

When one realizes that a single cell missed by the microscope may eventually form another aggressive tumor, the rationale for a rush to "curative" surgery becomes unclear. Further clouding the matter is the observation that at least 25% of breast cancers, 20% of malignant melanomas (deadly skin cancer) and 50% of prostate cancers tend to neither grow nor metastasize. A 2008 Canadian mammography study actually showed that 10% of proven breast cancers spontaneously disappeared over a 6-year study—by extension, might this not be true of prostate cancers, given the similarity between breast and prostate? The question for the patient becomes not, "How should I treat this?" but rather, "Should I defer a treatment decision and simply monitor this from time to time?" The wisdom of monitoring is bolstered by the growing awareness of an entity called "interval cancer." This is a class of rapidly growing, aggressive tumors that may arise spontaneously within weeks or months of a normal exam. The previous or ongoing treatment of a low grade tumor may give misplaced confidence to a patient who has just unknowingly developed a high grade tumor but doesn't think he needs further observation. To further complicate matters, autopsy studies on men dying from automobile accidents in Boston demonstrated prostate cancers in some men in their 30's. More alarming is the knowledge that many dangerous interval cancers do not cause PSA elevation and are mostly found in patients with low PSA levels. However, there's reason to hope: the Hattangadi study mentioned in the previous chapter showed that while this type of tumor may not announce itself via PSA, if it is detected by DRE when it is still focal, it is treatable. *We need to be alert to their existence.* Today's advanced imaging will undoubtedly make these tumors easier to identify earlier.

Prostate cancers have similarities to breast cancers in many aspects, since both organs are glands and their tissues look remarkably similar under the microscope. Autopsy data from a Harvard Medical school study of women dying from automobile accidents revealed 39% of women between the ages of forty to fifty years had breast cancer cells when only 1% of women would have been expected by usual clinical standards to have breast tumors. A multicenter mammogram study twenty years ago on Long Island women, where the breast cancer incidence is disproportionately high, showed that biopsies for malignant appearing calcifications on x-ray mammography revealed a greater percentage of microscopic cancers not in the areas suspected of being cancer, but rather in the unsuspected regions adjacent to the expected cancer sites. Another Harvard study presented to the New York Cancer Society at the 2009 Annual Meeting showed data demonstrating the breast tissue is continually developing both benign and malignant tumors. Most of these never become clinically significant. The message from these reports is: *many cancers are not lethal.*

Half a century ago, pathologists found that a high percentage of men without clinically demonstrated prostate cancer had malignant cells in the operative specimens from surgery for relief of benign prostatic obstruction. Without an evident tumor, perhaps cancer cells should be considered a nonthreatening aspect of normal body aging, or at worst, a chronic disease.

Blood flow: a detectable sign of tumor activity

Is there a way to determine whether a cancer is part of the natural aging process to be watched or whether the malignancy has potential deadly consequences, as with interval cancers? In 1985, a prominent British radiologist and physician, David Cosgrove, published a paper in the *American Journal of Radiology* demonstrating the presence of blood flows in breast cancers. After reading his article, I hopped on a plane and visited the Radiology Department at Hammersmith Hospital in London. There I observed the test first hand and envisioned future potential uses. I noted the new generation of sonogram equipment now had the capability to show pictures of blood vessels. The arteries and veins supplying a tumor could be clearly imaged. Moreover, the actual flowing blood in the cancer could be seen and the velocity of flow of blood in the vessels accurately measured. At an international conference in Italy in 1997, Dr. Rodolfo Campani, an Italian radiologist specializing in studying the blood flows of cancers at the University of Pavia Medical Center, identified the criteria to differentiate vessels supplying blood to malignancies from those attached to benign (noncancerous) tumors. Benign vessels are few in number, smoothly outlined, follow straight courses and branch regularly. Malignant vessels are many in number, irregularly outlined, irregular in course and crooked in branching patterns.

There are other blood velocity differences that are too technical for this book; however, it should be noted that malignant vessels have greater flow volumes at the end of the heart pumping cycle than benign vessels. These findings have been confirmed by other investigators at the 2012 World Congress of Interventional Oncology. Malignant blood vessels may be accurately and noninvasively detected by newer Doppler sonography techniques and advanced blood flow MRI protocols. Studies of tissue density or hardness have been perfected and also guide the assessment of tumor aggression. The harder or denser a tumor is, the more likely it is to be malignant. Ultrasound elastic measurements and MRI diffusion (hardness) data now quantify tumor aggression and are complementary with the blood flow technologies. This wealth of diagnostic input assists both patients and doctors in decision making.

Ultrasound and sonography

Sonograms use ultrasound. In fact, the terms are clinically identical. The physical principle of ultrasound, the piezoelectric effect where sound is created from electrical energy, was discovered by Pierre and Marie Curie 10 years before the recognition of the x-ray. The French military developed sonar to detect submarines during the First World War. Modern sonar was invented by American industrialists for checking metal flaws in railroad ties. It was later perfected by the US military for navigational use and underwater scanning. Early medical uses included imaging disorders of the eye, heart and the developing fetus. As computers grew in sophistication, so did the applications of ultrasound, and now it is often used as the first diagnostic test for many medical disorders. Doppler sonar created in 1972 gives pictures of flow movement in the human body in the same way it shows motion of storms and tornadoes in the weather patterns (Doppler radar) that one sees on television weather reports. Doppler technology has been around for years. One patient told me that he designed and built missiles for the US Army at the White Sands Proving Grounds in New Mexico in the 1950's. He related that the technique was so sensitive that it had to be continually modified and toned down; an air conditioner turned on a mile away could trigger a missile's detection system to arm and prepare to fire—once, a missile actually launched toward a moving train and followed it along the Santa Fe railroad tracks.

Urologists in Japan, oncologists in England, surgeons in the Netherlands, chemotherapists in Belgium, ultrasonographers in Scandinavia and radiologists in France, seeing the success of sonograms in diagnosing malignant tumors in the breast, turned their attention to the study of the prostate. They concluded that the vascular pattern shown by the Doppler technique held the key to the degree of malignancy. Ten years ago, German surgeons at the University of Ulm, the largest bone tumor center in Europe, showed that highly malignant bone cancers had high blood flows. The standard treatment for bone cancer is amputation of the entire limb. Bone tumors that demonstrate no vascularity or low blood flows are now watched or treated more conservatively. The current clinical use of this technique in Europe thus prevents unnecessary amputations.

Dr. Nathalie Lassau, an interventional radiologist at the Institute de Cancerologie Gustav Roussy, an internationally known cancer center in Paris, published similar findings on the deadly skin cancer, melanoma. Her article in the *American Journal of Radiology* in 2002 revealed lethal skin cancers to be highly vascular and skin cancers that could be watched were not vascular. Dr. Lassau is currently investigating medicines and performing curative treatments to reduce blood flows to cancers in hope of lessening their malignant consequences and has presented this work at numerous international meetings. Her finding that 3D Doppler sonography correlates best with the pathologic process was highlighted at the 2012 Journees Francaises de Radiologie Meeting in Paris. Newer MRI imaging protocols are currently being fine-tuned based on the proven high accuracy of the color and power of Doppler sonography data.

The blood flow patterns depicted by Doppler sonography provide a way to quantitatively measure and serially monitor the severity of malignancy throughout the treatment course. Blood flow analysis can reveal treatment response, since the size and number of tumor vessels decreases with successful therapies. Although this concept was described in the early 1990's in Europe, it was first mentioned in the American literature in 1996 at the American Roentgen Ray Society Annual Meeting. Dr. E. Louvar from Henry Ford Hospital (Detroit, MI) combined radiology and pathology studies to determine that the power Doppler flows in malignancies was correlated to the vessels that feed aggressive tumors. Significantly higher Gleason scores (more dangerous tumors described later) were seen in cancer biopsies of high Doppler flow areas compared to cancers with no Doppler flows. Dr. D. Downey at John Robarts Research Institute (University Hospital, Ontario, Canada) has looked at vascular imaging techniques and 3-D imaging of blood vessels. Blood vessels can be rendered in 3-D with angiography (high intensity dye injected into arteries), CT scanning (medium intensity dye), MR angiography (low intensity dye), Contrast Enhanced Ultrasound (low intensity dye not FDA approved), 3-D color Doppler imaging (no injection or dye) and 3-D power Doppler imaging (no injection or dye). In his article published in the *American Journal of Radiology* in 1995, he noted that power Doppler was better able to delineate abnormal vessel architecture in prostate cancers than color Doppler techniques. Since then we now use even more sensitive Doppler modalities with better computer analysis of tumor vessel concentrations.

Dr. Miroslav Zalesky, a urologist from Prague, Czechoslovakia delivered a paper at the 98th AUA Annual Meeting in Chicago (2003). He noted that blood vessels observed by the 3D PDS technology in the prostate determined extracapsular spread with 89% accuracy in a series of 282 patients. The spread of abnormal vessels from the gland through the capsule was highly significant and best demonstrated using the 3D capability for interpretation. Dr. Zalesky felt that 3D reconstruction enables physicians to biopsy areas of suspicious neovascularization (new abnormal arteries and veins) that would be missed by the standard sextant biopsy. In a response, Dr. Michael Brawer, a urologist not involved in the study, and quoted in the April 30th 2003 issue of *Doctor's Guide* on the internet, commented: "It is uncertain at this point whether the new modality can detect the fine vessels that are typical of the neovascularization found in cancer…The problem is that the size of the vessel delineated with Doppler is larger than the vessels found in malignancies. Are our imaging modalities sensitive enough to identify the small vessels characteristic of cancer? I don't know." While Dr. Brawer may be correct, he may also be missing the point that we do not need to see the small vessels associated with cancer to identify tumors, but can assume that growing malignancy needs nourishment by larger vessels easily seen on the Doppler to distribute blood to the smaller intratumor arteries.

Using Doppler technologies

A 2004 newsletter from the Prostate Cancer Research Institute reported that hormone therapy may change the way the pathologist interprets a cancer. A pathologist looks at a frozen anatomic picture of a cell which may or may not be indicative of the cells' current activity. For this reason, functional imaging using blood flow technologies assists in determining tumor aggression. Androgen deprivation therapy (ADT) makes it more difficult to grade the tumor with the microscope. Men who have been on ADT should have a Doppler sonogram study to confirm the absence of residual disease. If there are areas of abnormal blood vessels, biopsy may be considered. Many patients who have been treated for cancer accept the presence of abnormal blood flows as proof of recurrence and choose treatments accordingly without further biopsies. Most patients use the amount of decrease in number of the visible blood vessels to represent the degree of success. Dr. Pam Unger, a prostate cancer pathology specialist at Mount Sinai Hospital in New York, mentioned in a personal communication that radiation changes also caused difficulties in reading the microscopic slides. Furthermore, pathologists generally don't look for blood vessels, and thus do not routinely evaluate the vascular pattern in the specimens they interpret. Another problem with biopsy interpretation is the over-the-counter herbal medicine market. Many of the products for prostate health have some hormonal effects that shrink the prostate and improve symptoms. However, no one has determined if the pharmacologic properties of these alternative health treatments change the cells of the prostate to mimic cancer when the pathologist studies them under a glass slide. Today, one must also consider the possible toxic effects on the prostate of medicines and supplements made by foreign companies.

A 60-year old patient came to me who had been diagnosed via biopsy with high grade cancer. The biopsy was reviewed by several experts who agreed upon the serious nature of his problem. Unsatisfied, he had another urologist take a second biopsy, who confirmed his hopes that he indeed had a less malignant tumor. To settle the matter, he flew from southern California for clarification by my Doppler test. The use of the sonogram, though non-invasive, was invaluable in succinctly detecting the level of malignancy of the tumor. The blood flow sonogram showed the majority of the tumor to be low grade (without blood vessels), but a critically located region near the capsule was high grade (vascular) and was beginning to break through the capsule of the prostate where it could more easily metastasize. This was confirmed by MRI exam and later by surgery when the tumor was completely removed.

A 55-year old man came to me reluctantly because his biopsy was negative, but his PSA was steadily rising. He had a sextant biopsy in which three biopsy samples are taken from each side of the midline of the gland, one each at the base, the mid-gland and the apex (today's standard biopsy is more likely to include 10-14 needle samples rather than the earlier total of six). The cancer was centered in the midline where the biopsy never reached. Up to one third (25-30%) of cancers will be missed by routine biopsies, which is why we now image the cancer before the biopsy to target the tumor more accurately. It will confirm a need to biopsy, and increase its accuracy. It also saves diagnostic time; if a biopsy is performed prior to imaging, the damage and bleeding make an MRI difficult to interpret for up to four months of healing.

Another 70-year old man was told he had a high grade cancer. His sonogram revealed a small tumor measuring 4 mm (1/8 inch) that was set well in from the prostate capsule. He therefore decided to watch it and see if it grew. Six months later it had not grown. Twelve months later showed no growth. Eighteen months later there was still no change. He informed me that he is postponing his 24-month follow up scan because he is now traveling around the world.

A 52-year old from the Midwest had a PSA of 5 one year ago. Thirty-one biopsies failed to find cancer. Upon his visit to our center, a large anterior nonpalpable mass was clearly visible, and by then it had broken through the capsule. Ironically, his latest PSA had lowered to 3. Back home, his urologist persuaded him to be rebiopsied. This time a Gleason 4+3 was discovered.

A 50 year old from the South was referred for consultation about local cryosurgery (freezing). He had 18 biopsies showing Gleason 4+4 on the left and was considering HIFU or focal cryosurgery to maintain his potency. All his biopsies on the right were benign. Upon digital rectal examination, I felt a mass on the right and told him so. "Doctor", he said, "the biopsy shows a tumor on the left, the right is normal." Upon seeing the large mass of abnormal blood vessels on the right and the penetration of the tumor through the right capsule and the comparatively few abnormal vessels on the left, he agreed to have an MRI exam. The special computerized MRI study confirmed bilateral tumors. He decided to try HIFU as a first line treatment as he and his young wife were intent upon expanding their family. They were relieved that the tumor on the left was not as aggressive on the scans as the biopsy indicated and that they were choosing a bilateral treatment instead of a focal one-sided therapy.

Medical progress and government regulation

In 1999 at the University of California San Diego, a French medical student, Dr. Olivier Lucidarme developed a highly sensitive technique to improve Doppler ultrasound. Special bubbles injected intravenously greatly improved imaging of small vessels. To date, our FDA has not approved this technology and Dr. Lucidarme now practices this methodology in Paris. Italian researchers Drs. Vito Cantisani and Francesco Drudi have demonstrated that this technology can show cancers unsuspected by other means. Advanced MRI scans performed in Europe are not available in the US, nor are certain sophisticated radioactive bone scans allowed in the states at this writing.

In addition to government approval processes, other factors influence which treatment a doctor may recommend to a patient. If you have an ulcer, an internist will give you pills, a psychiatrist will offer psychotherapy and a surgeon will recommend an operation. The cancer treatment field likewise provides a host of traditional and nontraditional options.

I do not recommend one treatment over another, since it is up to the patient to study all possibilities before discussing them with his treating physician. However, doing diligent research can result in frustration when a patient learns of a promising treatment—only to find out it's not available in his own country! A case in point is the early detection of metastatic cancer lesions. Metastases is the most dreaded word for patients since it indicates their primary tumor has spread to remote parts of their body and hope for a cure is lost. In 2004, my colleague, Dr. Jelle Barentsz, head of Cancer Research at Nijmegen University Hospital in Holland, presented a paper at the International Congress of Radiology in which he described a new technique to evaluate cancer spreading to the lymph nodes. It uses MRI with a novel contrast agent called Combidex and the technique is termed MRL (Magnetic Resonance Lymphangiography.) This technology is extremely important since MRI is the best way to image abnormal nodes that are hidden or inaccessible at surgery. The imaging shows the size and location of the lymph nodes as well as the presence of cancerous tissue as small as 1/5 inch. This critical piece of information that pinpoints cancer infiltration tells where the spread occurs and allows for accurate treatment planning. The current "gold standard" for lymph node evaluation is surgery called *pelvic lymph node dissection.* Clearly this invasive exploratory operation, where the surgeon searches with his hand for hard lumps in the abdomen, cannot find all the tiny disease sites to which cancer spreads. The MRL exam is so accurate that a negative exam translates into a 96% chance that there is no metastatic disease to the lymph nodes. In addition to sparing patients from the risk and pain of surgery, this methodology reduces health care costs. So why was the test not approved in France in 2008 and yet to be approved in the US? Ask your congressman why you have to go to the Netherlands to see if your cancer has spread!

CHAPTER 4

PRACTICAL ANATOMY, PATHOLOGY AND DIAGNOSIS

Only as you know yourself can your brain
serve you as a sharp and efficient tool.
—**Bernard Baruch**

U rologic anatomy highlights the strategic benefits of the newer technologies:

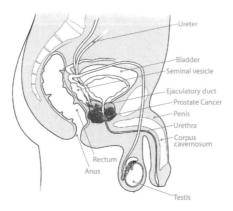

Fig. 4.1 Anatomy of male pelvic area showing
aggressive prostate cancer and nearby structures

Important anatomic zones are the **base** of the prostate (next to the bladder), the **apex** (farthest from the bladder) and the **mid-gland** (between the base and the apex). Like an avocado, the gland has an outer zone called the peripheral zone in which most cancers occur and a central zone (similar to the avocado pit) where 20% of cancers occur, and the growths that develop there are usually benign. The nerves that are necessary for erection lie along the gland on both right and left sides of the exterior of the prostate capsule; because the nerves are "bundled" with very small blood vessels, these structures are called **neurovascular bundles.**

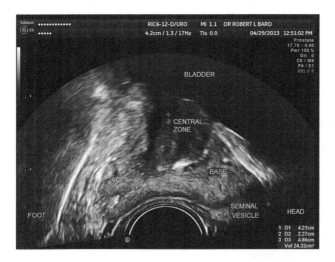

Fig. 4.2 Ultrasound anatomy of prostate

What is PSA and can it reveal prostate cancer?

The PSA test, which stands for Prostate Specific Antigen, was first used in the criminal justice system to determine if a woman was raped. PSA is a type of enzyme secreted by epithelial cells in the prostate gland. The PSA blood test measures how much of the antigen is contained in blood or semen. Thus, the test was not originally designed to indicate cancer; if a woman's vaginal fluid was PSA positive, then that positively indicated male semen.

The usual test is called Total PSA. There also exist variations: Free PSA, Complex PSA, bPSA, iPSA and proPSA. Free PSA is often elevated due to benign problems. Complex PSA appears more specific for cancer. PSAV (PSA Velocity changes over time) is proving more useful. Men must be aware that these variations exist so they can make accurate comparisons. Patients must also realize that the increasing number of modifiers of this screening modality attest to its lack of specificity.

Lectures at the 2006 AUA Meeting by Dr. D'Amico and colleagues showed that men with a PSAV greater than 1.8 ng/ml per year had a higher incidence of Gleason 7, 8, 9 and 10 tumors.

When the PSA blood test was devised in the 1980s as a possible way to screen for prostate cancer, normal levels were considered to be 0-4.0 ng/ml, and anything above that was considered grounds for a biopsy. Its use in this fashion has often rushed men into a needle biopsy, a questionable practice when imaging is now widely available to validate whether or not an invasive biopsy is warranted. Other factors besides prostate cancer can elevate PSA blood levels. A large study from Boston five years ago showed that the test underestimated the presence of cancer in two thirds of those examined and overestimated the likelihood of cancer in two thirds of the patients. Explanations that erroneous levels are due to prostatitis, or a previous biopsy, or a large gland, or inflammation or even a recent ejaculation are useful only in theory. A 2004 report from the Memorial Sloan Kettering Cancer Center, published in the prestigious *Journal of the American Medical Association*, reported that a man's PSA levels fluctuate naturally over time, which leads to false elevated scores. To add to the controversy, a paper published by Dr. Ian Thompson (University of Texas Health Science Center, San Antonio) in *The New England Journal of Medicine* (May 2004) reported his study of 2,940 men aged 62-79. He found that as many as 15% with "normal" PSA levels less than 4 ng/ml had cancer when assessed by biopsies.

Concerned about the uncertainties of PSA levels as a useful indication of potential cancer, and the potential threat of slow growing cancers, physicians and patients all too frequently opt to remove the entire prostate gland as a precaution. According to a 2004 article by Dr. Thomas Stamey of Stanford University in California, researchers at Stanford have concluded that a full 98% of all prostates removed at their medical center over the past five years were done so unnecessarily. Only 2% warranted removal due to cancers large enough to cause concern. This surprising result validates the findings of Stamey and others that elevated PSA blood levels occur naturally as aging prostate glands enlarge naturally, and thus are not a definitive cancer marker.

In the absence of a perfect modality for detecting cancerous cells in the prostate, there is another standard test. The digital rectal exam (DRE) uses the examiner's finger to find hard regions in the gland. Firm areas that are nodular and irregular usually indicate moderately advanced cancer. However, postoperative or postbiopsy scarring of the prostate, tuberculosis (TB), sarcoidosis (glandular disorder like TB) and stones in this organ may simulate a tumor, resulting in an ambiguous DRE. In addition, this exam only checks the outside of the prostate and does miss growths on the side and in the deeper (anterior) regions that lie distant and out of reach of the probing examiner's finger. While there is value to the DRE in detecting a subset of tumors (interval cancers) that don't express PSA, it too is not perfect by any means.

Dr. William Pitts, in an article in the 2003 *British Journal of Urology*, feels that PSA is only of worth in detecting recurrence following surgical removal. Other researchers agree that a measurable and rising PSA in a man with an irradiated or surgically removed prostate probably indicates a new malignancy local site or in the adjacent lymph nodes and bones. As more experience is gained with postoperative patients using combined MRI and ultrasound scans, physicians are finding that patients without local recurrence may still have measurable PSA levels that, in part, may be due to the spread of cancer to distant sites or may be due to inherent inaccuracies in the test itself. Many physicians, however, still believe that a slowly and steadily rising PSA level indicates a true malignancy.

Dr. Len Lichtenfeld, Deputy Chief Medical Officer at the American Cancer Society, admits that there are no easy answers. He recognizes that even a man with a low PSA may harbor a microscopic, asymptomatic tumor, and as such favors screening and biopsy. He acknowledges, "We will find more prostate cancer, and we will find more cancers that didn't need to be found. We will cause some men harm that they didn't need to have." Dr. Gilbert Welch, a professor of medicine at the Department of Veterans Affairs, says men should consider whether they want a PSA test at all. He said, "It is becoming increasingly clear that the more pathologists look for cancer, the more they will find it, but that does not mean the cancer is worth finding." The 2011 British Medical Association and the 2012 American Medical Society both recommend giving patients the option of PSA testing.

The EPCA test

Dr. Robert Getzenberg, director of urologic research at Johns Hopkins University School of Medicine, in the 2007 journal *Urology*, described a new blood test that may replace the PSA as a screening tool. He notes the test is for a protein found only in the nucleus or prostate cancer cells and is called "early prostate cancer antigen-2 or EPCA-2" This is not found in normal cells.

When it enters the blood stream, it remains for a long time and can be measured on a screening basis. Apparently, the levels in the serum can differentiate between organ confined tumor and cancer that has spread beyond the gland. The false positive rate was 3%, meaning no cancer was found when the test indicated a tumor. The false negative percentage was 6%, meaning cancer was found when the test diagnosed no tumor. He noted the specificity of the exam may distinguish between benign disease (BPH and prostatitis) and reduce the estimated 1.3 million to 1.6 million men undergoing yearly biopsies to identify the 230,000 patients with cancer.

All the more reason to employ imaging

As an early pioneer in the use of PSA to diagnose prostate cancer, Dr. Stamey's views on its use are significant. It is noteworthy that he is rethinking the use of PSA readings when considering options for prostate cancer detection and treatment. While PSA elevation is normal with aging, any PSA blood test above ten is a reason for a biopsy. However, Dr. Stamey's team of researchers is looking for a more accurate way to determine the presence and severity of cancer in the prostate. Currently, they are working on a blood test that relates to the size of the tumor, but as yet have met with little success. Remember, the most virulent cancers (called *anaplastic* tumors or interval cancers) do not produce sufficient PSA to reflect in elevated values. This means the worst malignancies may have the lowest PSA numbers. This also means the more accurate sonogram and MRI technology should be considered to replace this blood test.

Gleason grading numbers and prognosis

Tumor grade refers to the microscopic appearance of cancer tissue obtained after biopsy or surgery and is named for the 1966 inventor, Dr. Donald Gleason. The Prostate Cancer Research Institute Newsletter of 2002 states only ten laboratories in the United States are accurate in their interpretation of the Gleason Score (GS or Gleason Sum) which determines the invasiveness of cancers. The Prostate Cancer Research Institute Newsletter of 2006 notes that pathologists have changed their grading patterns to higher numbers over the last decade and there is ongoing discussion of changing the methodology to more clearly represent significant disease. Indeed, pathologists have acknowledged that the numbers from biopsies are often upgraded or downgraded when the actual gland is surgically removed and examined by microscopic sections.

Tumor grading is defined as a property of cancer independent of tumor location found in either a biopsy or operative specimen. Grading is based on the appearance of biopsied cells, and is up to the judgment of the pathologist examining them. The more they appear like normal cells, the lower the score—but the more disorganized and chaotic, the higher the score. Scores range from 1-5 per sample, and are always based on two samples: primary and secondary.

The GS primary grade is the most important pattern that the pathologist sees in the tumor under the microscope and must be greater than 50% of the total pattern. The secondary grade is the next most predominant pattern and must be at least 5% of the total pattern. The Gleason score is the sum of both patterns observed. The GS is always shown as a sum of two numbered specimens (with the predominant score listed first). Summed scores range from 2-10 with 10 indicating the most malignant. For instance, a patient might learn that his positive biopsy received a GS of 3+3, equal to a total GS of 6. Note that there is a difference between GS 4+3 = 7 and GS 3+4 = 7. Although they both equal 7, the 4+3 score indicates a more aggressive disease than 3+4, because the 4 was the primary score, or larger of the two samples. Newer investigation techniques used by modern pathologists are now showing that many cases of GS = 2 cancer were actually an abnormal benign growth (adenosis) which mimics cancers but is not actually malignant. In current practice, a Gleason 6 (3+3) or lower may be considered a low grade tumor whereas a higher number is generally more malignant. While prognosis or survival is often correlated with Gleason score, perhaps a better indicator would be the image-monitored response of a tumor's vascularity to the current treatment regimen.

It is important to understand that biopsies guided by transrectal ultrasound (TRUS biopsies) may be random and sometimes difficult to interpret. One reason I attended the Armed Forces Institute of Pathology was to learn the discrepancy between what the microscopic analysis predicted and the actual outcome. It appears that how biopsy tissue appears under the microscope is best correlated with the imaging findings on x-rays, CT, MRI, PET and ultrasound studies. Such cross-referencing was particularly valuable in bone cancers, since the microscopic picture of a healing fracture is almost identical to a serious malignancy. I also recall Dr. Jack Rabinowitz, Chief of Radiology at my residency program at The Brooklyn Hospital (and later Chief of Radiology at Mount Sinai Medical Center in New York) in 1970 showing a surgeon that his working diagnosis of bone cancer was unsupported by the radiologic findings suggesting lymphoma (gland cancer) metastatic to the bone. The surgeon reviewed the case, decided against operating to amputate the leg, and the patient was successfully treated medically instead of surgically. Extending these illustrations to clinical work with prostate tumors, there are significant implications for diagnosis and treatment decisions. It makes perfect sense that the information from 3-D color Doppler sonograms can overcome the shortcomings of PSA, DRE and TRUS biopsies.

Magnetic Resonance Imaging (MRI) of the prostate

MRI refers to the image of signal intensity in the gland with the patient in the tube of the unit. There are several MRI formats for examining the prostate:

a) EC-MRI (Endorectal Coil MRI) uses a wand-like coil inserted within an inflatable balloon into the rectum to improve resolution in the prostate.

b) S-MRI (Spectroscopic MRI) involves analysis of the chemical composition of the prostate tissues with emphasis on the compound *choline.*

c) DCE-MRI (Dynamic Contrast Enhanced MRI) uses the injection of a contrast agent *gadolinium* that reveals the blood flow within tumorous prostatic tissue. 3.0 Tesla (higher strength) and DCE-MRI also referred to as Full Time Point (FTP) DCE-MRI will be discussed in a later chapter.[2]

MRI shows cancer as a loss or decrease of the normal glandular prostatic tissue signal; however, other benign pathologies, such as calculi, hemorrhage (bleeding from recent biopsy), stones, BPH and inflammation may also produce this effect. Some infiltrating types of cancer will not produce any visible changes. The data from the 2009 American Roentgen Ray Meeting shows a 75% sensitivity (25% false negatives) and 95% specificity (5% false positives). MRI was originally used to stage the spread of cancer outside the prostate gland known as ECE (extra capsular extension). The data showed ECE medium specificity (74%) and sensitivity (71%).

EC-MRI using the endorectal coil inflated as a balloon was designed to better define the capsule of the gland and the seminal vesicles. However, they have other difficulties since they tend to migrate upwards into the looser and

---

2   The reader may wish to purchase a textbook titled *DCE MRI Of Prostate Cancer* (Springer Publishing, 2009) written by myself. I am now Editor in Chief of *Image Guided Prostate Cancer Treatments* to be published in 2014.

wider part of the bowel rather than remain fixed where the prostate narrows the rectum. This results in degraded images of the apex (the part of the prostate closer to the narrow anus). Physicians have observed image distortion or deforming due to the flattening of the rectal border of the prostate by the endorectal coil. Additionally, the endorectal coil with its balloon is by uncomfortable, promoting more patient motion and degrading the exam results. The stiller the patient remains and quieter the patient's insides, the better the MRI images turn out. Lastly, the coil's pressure may cause dilation of the intraprostatic urethra or abnormal kinking and narrowing, rendering diagnosis of these conditions more difficult. My practice has optimal results without using an endorectal coil as long as the DCE-MRI is simultaneously compared with the sonographic findings.

S-MRI was designed to detect intraglandular cancer and show the aggression. The spectroscopic chemical analysis of cancer shows higher levels of proteins (choline and citrate) than in normal prostatic tissues. The analyzed sections of the prostate are divided into a grid pattern of such a size that small cancers could be missed. While this technique appeared useful for larger tumors, a 2005 *Radiology* journal article noted an overall sensitivity of 56% for tumor detection. Currently S-MRI is practiced at few medical centers in the US and is losing popularity at many international academic facilities. A 2012 presentation by Dr. O. Rouviere from Lyon, France at the French Radiology Meeting highlighted the problem that S-MRI was not effective in analyzing tumor extension into the fatty tissues adjacent to the prostate gland.

DCE-MRI is widely used and has improved specificity by about 80% according to the 2008 *Radiology* article by Drs. J. Futterer and J. Barentsz and sponsored by the Dutch Cancer Society. This group has developed a 3-D S-MRI system that improves the overall accuracy of standard S-MRI.

An MRI exam shows the extent of cancer but not the activity. In patients successfully treated by hormones, the abnormality may still persist on the MRI picture, whereas the Doppler test has the advantage of showing blood flows that are greatly reduced or completely absent. S-MRI, also designed to show activity, has not been shown to be as sensitive as physicians had hoped. Indeed, one physician colleague, who flew from New York City to San Francisco for this test, was told the S-MRI showed extensive cancer; subsequently, 12 biopsied samples revealed no cancer. At the 2004 meeting of the New York Roentgen Society devoted to prostate cancer, Dr. Steven Eberhardt (Memorial Sloan

Kettering Cancer Center) said that S-MRI was inaccurate in the presence of prostatitis because it produced false positive results. He went on to clarify the pro's and con's of regular MRI with the use of an endorectal coil, mentioning that evaluation of the base is difficult due to the normal variation of anatomy of the prostate. Benign prostatic hypertrophy, commonly called BPH, often distorts the peripheral zone, the most common site for cancer. Also, stones and hemorrhage (bleeding) from biopsies, and variations of the central prostatic zonal (internal) anatomy, could simulate cancers. Dr. Jelle O. Barentsz, Chair of Research, at the University Medical Center Nijmegen, Netherlands, said that S-MRI results would be inaccurate following androgen deprivation therapy (hormone therapy, Chinese herbs, PC-SPES, etc.) and disagreed that prostatitis was a problem.[3] The consensus at the 2012 JFR Meeting was this: S-MRI would be discontinued if the new generation of MRI units (3 Tesla with twice the strength of the standard 1.5 Tesla units) did not provide more accurate results.

Another problem with MRI exams is the variation of normal anatomy and the changes in the prostate formed by the commonplace benign enlargement called benign prostatic hypertrophy also known as benign prostatic hyperplasia (BPH). It has been widely acknowledged that the internal anatomy of the prostate may vary from individual to individual. It was becoming obvious that benign enlargement made MRI exams more difficult for physicians in this field to interpret. However, it was assumed that the capsule of tissue that held and contained the gland and also prevented spread of the tumor to regions outside the prostate was regular. It was shown in 2004 in the *American Journal of Radiology* that there is a normal irregularity to the capsule of the prostate in about 10% of men. This is surprising news to the imaging medical community and deserves further study. Unfortunately, the finding of capsular irregularity has been one of the cardinal signs for spread of the cancer in the prostate. Fortunately, the latest generation of ultrasound probes has a resolution 5 times greater than the MRI and can verify capsule integrity.

After I gave a 2012 Mt. Sinai Symposium lecture on ultrasound imaging of malignant melanoma, a lady dermatologist came up to me and asked if this could diagnose prostate cancer. Her husband was reluctant to be tested. A few days later,

---

3   Dr. Barentz solved the problem of endorectal coil movement by injections (glucagons) to paralyze the colon for a full hour to complete the entire exam. One of my older patients, who had visited Dr. Barentsz in Holland, wryly observed that he did not have a normal bowel movement following the exam until 96 hours later.

she brought him into my office for an examination. He said his urologist had found some enlargement but nothing suspicious. My DRE (digital rectal exam) revealed a large mass that was palpable but not very hard. The sonogram instantly showed an 18 mm (1/2 inch) tumor in the area where I felt it. The tumor was very well circumscribed, rounded and avascular. It did not look like a cancer. In fact, 5% of BPH nodules that usually form in the central zone can occur in the peripheral zone. That was his happy ending.

Looking for signs of cancer

In diagnosing tumors physicians look for a dominant mass, a tumor bulge and loss of the normal internal prostatic architecture (usually in the peripheral zone). The 2004 International Congress of Radiology in Montreal noted that only 15% of urologists use any form of MRI to evaluate the prostate and that use is generally to see if the tumor has spread to the adjacent glands. Unlike urologists, radiologists were early proponents of prostate applications for MRI. Dr. H. Mao, a radiologist at the Emory University in Atlanta, suggested, in the 2005 issue of *Diagnostic Imaging*, that the latest version of the MRI (called 3T MRI) is not only useful for monitoring and staging prostate cancer, but "would recommend it for screening if it could be comfortable and affordable, since it shows the prostate structure so clearly."

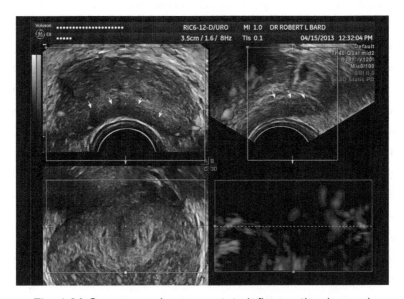

Fig. 4.3A Sonogram shows prostate inflammation (arrows)

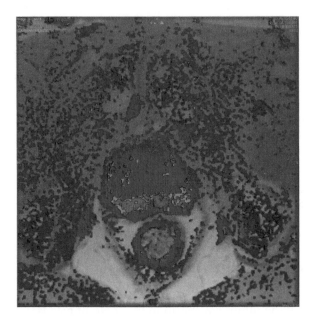

Fig. 4.3B MRI shows inflammation as red area

Sonography of the prostate

I started examining the prostate thirty-nine years ago with equipment that took sonograms from the skin surface on the lower part of the abdomen over a full urinary bladder. These were termed "transabdominal" pelvic sonograms. Nineteen years ago, probes were developed to insert into the rectum, providing better images by placing the tip closer to the prostate. This development was called "transrectal ultrasound" or TRUS.

Twelve years ago I worked with urologists performing prostate biopsies under ultrasound guidance (TRUS biopsies). I would scan the prostate and tell the surgeon the suspicious area to biopsy. The Doppler blood flows have proven to be the best indicator of highly malignant tumors as a region of high flow is 450% more likely to have a positive biopsy result. The American College of Radiology uses the blood flow density as an indicator for the best area to biopsy, as stated in the 2004 edition of *The Standards of the American College of Radiology*. Nine years ago, the Austrians perfected 3-D imaging of the prostate which allowed physicians to optimally visualize the outer capsule of the prostate. This is a particularly important border since the spread of cancer outside the capsule means it is no longer operable. At the International Congress of Radiology in 2004, Dr. David Cosgrove, a leading English authority of color and power Doppler ultrasound imaging, voiced his approval of the use of this technology to determine the aggressiveness of prostate cancers. In 2013, Dr. Cosgrove presented a new study at the American Institute of Ultrasound (AIUM) meeting. He had been testing a new ultrasound modality that shows hardness of tumors and is 99% accurate in detecting breast tumors. This exam is called *elastography*, is still under study for use in the prostate.

The prostate capsule

Much emphasis has been placed by patients and physicians on extension of cancer outside the fibrous covering of the prostate gland. This so-called extracapsular extension (ECE) was supposed to mean the cancer is inoperable and presumably fatal in the long term. Noted earlier in the book, pathology studies have shown that MRI depiction of this entity is at best 90% accurate. More important, clinically localized cancers are proven to lie outside the prostate at least 50% of the time. Dr. Stylianos Lomvardias, a urologic pathologist formerly at the AFIP (Armed Forces Institute of Pathology) has described normal prostate glands in the muscle outside the prostate borders. Surgeons often find the capsule difficult to visualize during the operation. Dr. Robert O'Connor, a urologic pathologist from the University Hospital in Ireland, has also attested to the fact that the so called capsule is often difficult to demonstrate in the post-operative specimen.

Perhaps the focus of treatment should be the location of the cancer in or out of the prostate gland and the invasiveness as demonstrated by 3D PDS rather than the "sentence" of inoperability when it has spread beyond the elusive capsular wall.

Two major presentations at the 2007 AUA meeting discussed the accuracy of imaging the prostatic capsule. A multicenter study from Harvard and the Medical College of Georgia looked at EC-MRI (endorectal MRI) in determining pre-operatively the status of the prostate capsule. Sixty two patients had radical prostatectomies with special attention to ECE (extracapsular extension). Eighty percent of T1C (clinically localized) cancers had positive margins at the operative pathologic review. The conclusion was EC-MRI was not valid in assessing ECE in prostate cancer. A larger study from the Medical University Innsbruck of 180 patients using 3D PDS showed 84% sensitivity, 96% specificity and an overall accuracy of 92% in detecting ECE. Furthermore, the positive predictive value (number of expected ECE cases) was 94% and the negative predictive value (number of expected non-ECE margins) was 91%.

Of greatest interest was the 90% accuracy in detecting seminal vesicle invasion. The authors concluded that 3D PDS is an accurate technique for staging localized prostate cancer, and, in the case of advanced disease, the detection of capsular perforation and seminal vesicle invasion was high.

While many men may be reluctant to avail themselves of current modalities detecting cancer in the prostate, an exam may ease the mind of a patient who believes he has cause for concern, and allay some unnecessary or irrational fears. A negative test alone would provide a significant comfort zone if done using highly accurate imaging. A positive test without detected blood flow means that a tumor is of a less aggressive nature, indicating that it will grow slowly. This is critical knowledge for men choosing watchful waiting, conservative management (lifestyle changes), or alternative treatments.

Although the sonogram test of the prostate may take different forms, they all use ultrasound high frequency waves and sophisticated computer analysis. It is a simple exam. Harmless sound waves ensure that the test is safe (no x-rays or radiation). It is rapid because of high technology imaging products. It is accurate, employing state-of-the-art computer reconstruction. Generally, the small lubricated probe is placed inside the rectum, although it may be applied to the perineum (area between the penis and anus) to obtain images if the rectal approach is not possible due to previous surgery. The probe has a wide field of vision, so there is very little movement involved. The sonographic physician or specially trained imaging technician looks at the instantaneous video appearing on the screen, taking pictures and measuring images according to a standard protocol, and notes and documents abnormalities. Two dimensional pictures are taken in "real time" which are similar to the images of the inside the pregnant mother's womb showing moving babies or the fetal heart beating. The 3-D or three-dimensional technology that shows the face of the baby is now successfully applied to the prostate. It is faster, yet it contains more information than the standard 2-D sonogram. Essentially, the 3-D machine takes a volume of pictures and stores this data inside the unit's computer banks. The data may be analyzed immediately or later reviewed and reconstructed in various angles or planes. In comparing 2-D with 3-D imaging, one can say the sonographer looks and then takes pictures with the 2-D system; whereas, with the 3-D technology pictures are taken which are then looked at and formally evaluated later. If a significant problem is seen and annotated with the 2-D exam, it cannot be later observed except by completely re-scanning the patient. The 3-D rendition may be reviewed over and over without recalling and re-examining the patient. 3-D imaging has made exam time shorter, providing more patient comfort. The images are then analyzed on a special computer work station allowing optimal rendering of the prostate in multiple planes as required.

An important variation of the 3-D is called 4-D, which adds the element of time to the exam and is used for the advanced image guided treatments described later in this book. While the 3-D sonogram takes only minutes to perform, 25 volume scans are performed every second in 3-D planes resulting in about 1,000 images that need to be reviewed and interpreted. Of the many technical features of 3-D imaging, "automatic acquisition" makes this test equivalent to an MRI or CT scan of the prostate, as it is multi-planar (in 3 planes) and accurately reproducible for comparison with an earlier or later study. The electronic array inside the probe sweeps back and forth, like a fan, over the prostate gland. A set of raw electronic data is stored in the sonogram memory that can be manipulated and studied as required at any time. The primary diagnostic breakthrough of 3-D/4-D imaging is to show visual "slices" of the prostate that see the capsule (outer margins) in what is called a coronal view.

This special view, available only on 3-D equipment, allows one to see invasion of cancer more easily. Specifically, the spread of cancer outside the prostate gland or ECE is well seen with this technique. This is critical clinical information, since ECE changes the cancer from operable to inoperable. The patient's own vascular pattern that determines aggression can be overlaid on the 3-D scan, which adds greatly to the assessment of the disease and the feasibility of treatment possibilities. This is notably useful in men with low-grade cancers who wish to be monitored during watchful waiting or alternative therapies thereby deferring whole gland treatment. Most low grade tumors remain localized and may be watched or controlled with noninvasive or minimally invasive treatments. The standard MRI cannot demonstrate tumor aggression in the moment, although comparisons from previous exams show progress and interval changes.

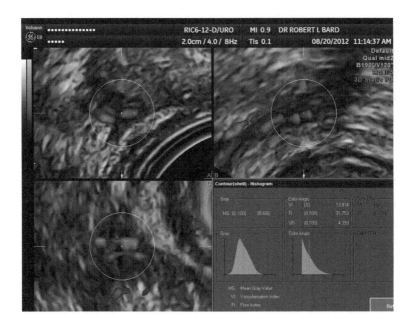

Fig. 4.4A Doppler shows 14% tumor vessel density (high)

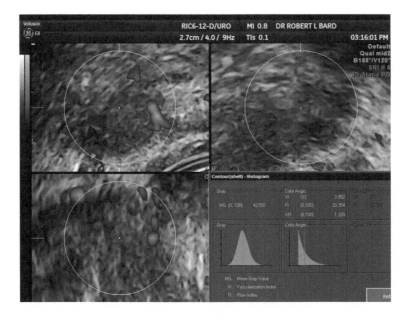

Fig. 4.4B Doppler shows vessel density decreased to 4% (post treatment)

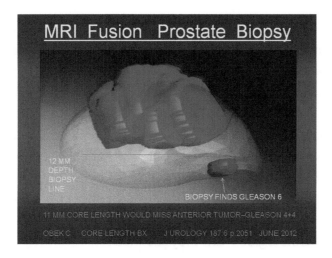

Fig. 4.5 Digital rectal exam and standard biopsy missed high grade tumor

Dr. Deborah Rubens, Associate Chair of Radiology and Surgery at the University of Rochester Medical Center, said in the January 2005 edition of *Diagnostic Imaging*, "With volume imaging, you're assured of getting everything you need. It standardizes exams, while providing us with new information and a new way to look at things." Dr. Rubens added that volumetric imaging is especially helpful when looking for multiple tumors or nodules. Since each region must be measured in several planes, it is easy to lose track of which nodule is which. She says that, "If you have them in a volume, you can just scroll through it. The next time that person comes in, it's easy to compare each problem area to what it looked like in the previous visit."

For example, a 65-year old California man had treated his Gleason 3+3 (low grade) tumor by macrobiotic lifestyle and naturopathic remedies that successfully controlled the cancer for five years. He was monitored in my office every six months, and there was no interval change demonstrated. On his 11th semiannual check up, I felt a firm mass during the DRE. The color flashed red on the computer screen, and we saw abnormal vessels. The 3D PDS (3-D power Doppler sonography) imaging showed the blood vessels penetrating through the capsule. The MRI exam later that day confirmed a large area of low grade cancer (Gleason 3+3) which remained unchanged and had not broken out of the prostate. However, where the new blood vessels appeared on the sonogram, the MRI revealed that there was a rupture in the capsule and new tumor penetration outside the prostate. After his initial disappointment, the patient realized that this red flag had probably saved his life by demonstrating a fresh and probably different type of cancer than the low grade tumor he had successfully treated for years with herbal supplements. He left our office a sobered but grateful person. Medical practitioners are realizing that the new entity called "interval cancer" appears more dangerous than the known cancers in both men and women. In this patient's case, a six month screening paid off as he knew he had alternate treatment options to choose. Dr. Robert Knapp, Professor Emeritus at Harvard Medical School and inventor of the CA125 blood test for cancer detection, described "interval cancers as the most virulent of prostate cancers that typically show up between screening examinations."

Screening technologies – are they justified?

One must look at existing cancer screening technologies and results to determine if significant disease is conclusively demonstrated. When I was a resident in training in 1970, everyone sought a yearly chest x-ray. Routine chest x-rays were eventually phased out because the yield of a true clinical problem was extraordinarily low. The *Journal of the American Medical Association* (January 2004) noted that 38% of asymptomatic screened adults experienced false positive findings, and half of those with abnormal results found the experience "very scary." The October 2011 recommendations by the US Government Panel to discontinue routine PSA screening for otherwise healthy men were based in part by a concern that PSA does not conclusively demonstrate significant disease, in part by a rush to invasive biopsies, and (if the biopsy were positive) a rush to whole gland treatments with the risk of urinary and sexual side effects. Knowing that PSA is a flawed tool, the Panel's conclusion is understandable.

The prostate sonogram done with advanced equipment by an experienced practitioner is a game-changer. We have an accurate, cost-effective way to screen for tumors and their degree of aggressiveness. In my practice of screening men for prostate cancer with sonograms, my colleagues and I have been surprised to find that about 5% of men with low or normal PSA had non-palpable aggressive cancers missed by clinical palpation. Now that sonogram screening for breast cancer has become as routine as the mammogram for women, it is logical to think that a non-invasive sonogram prostate screening modality may supplant the currently used PSA and DRE. Perhaps this will be named similar to the woman's mammogram and be called the men's screening "prostagram" or "prostasound."

There are, of course, possible errors with sonogram investigations. The regular 2-D sonogram may miss low grade cancers that have the same appearance as the normal gland, which account for up to 40% of prostate tumors, according to Dr. D. Downey (*Urology 1997*). The overall accuracy is about 50%. The accuracy is better in glands that have never been subjected to a biopsy or treated in any way. The accuracy is lower in prostates that have been biopsied multiple times or in persons who have been treated with radiation or hormones. The power Doppler study adds about 30% more accuracy, since the abnormal blood vessels provide a road map to the tumor; however, detours on the road may occur in the presence of inflammation, stones or calculi. Indeed, a US patent (No. 5,860,929) was obtained by Norwegian scientists to determine power Doppler blood flows in optimally diagnosing prostate cancers. When a stone is identifiable, the sound waves bounce back so strongly that they create a false color pattern. This pattern to the trained clinician will not be mistaken for a tumor vessel. Fortunately, the Doppler technology has other formats that correctly identify the artifactual or spurious colors, distinguishing it from a true cancer. In my practice, combining 3D PDS with focused computer aided vascular MRI exams, we have achieved a 97% overall accuracy in diagnosing and staging prostate cancers. An important exception occurs in the seminal vesicles, which sit on top of the prostate gland generating the fluid that produces the ejaculation. Early cancer spread to these paired vesicles may be missed by the 3D PDS. When a tumor is found near or adjacent to the seminal vesicles at the base of the prostate, MRI scans are mandatory. MRI technology may also assist in differentiating inflammation from tumor vessels.

Applying sonograms to prostate cancer treatments

Japanese investigators, Osamu Ukimura and Tsuneharu Miki, studied the use of 3D PDS in nerve sparing surgery, and presented their findings at the 2005 AUA Meeting. Using European ultrasound systems during laparoscopic radical prostatectomy (LRP or robot guided surgical removal of the prostate) they were able to visualize the nerves of the prostate and protect them during surgery. This improved outcomes in terms of potency and continence. It also improved surgical margins meaning less volume of tumor was left behind. The real time imaging also showed the surgeon unsuspected tumors that were outside the planned operative field in 44% of patients in the study. This alerted the surgeon to make a wider incision to include the newly discovered tumor. The authors also noted that injury to the adjacent rectal wall and bladder neck was avoided since these areas were continuously monitored. They concluded, "Real time TRUS during LRP can map important periprostatic structures and any clinically significant cancer nodules, potentially enhancing the precision of the laparoscopic procedure." Needless to say, improving surgical outcomes with fewer side effects, thanks to ultrasound, is a gift to men.

CHAPTER 5

TRUST EXPERIENCE
AND GATHER INFORMATION

In 1996, Dr. Michael Schachter, a prominent alternative medicine practitioner called me and asked me if I would like to learn a new treatment protocol for my patients. This new treatment was from a patient who had successfully regressed his own cancer. Dr. Schachter told me that he had developed his own effective alternative medical therapy protocols based on experience gained from the successes and failures of his own patients. Dr. Schachter introduced me to Larry Clapp, who convinced me that his naturopathic healing had worked. When Larry allowed me to scan his biopsy proven high grade Gleason tumor, I saw all that remained was a scar. This meant a healed, inactive area had taken the place of a deadly cancer. When Larry told me that cancer was not a disease but a reactive response to a body disturbed by toxins and hormonal imbalance, I began to listen. As a formally trained radiologist, the thought of cancer not being *de facto* a disease didn't make sense; however, I was faced with the incontrovertible fact of a malignancy killed without drugs, radiation or surgery. As a physician trained in traditional medicine, this remarkable observation sparked my interest. Since then, I have listened to my patients carefully and

53

garnered experience with a wide collection of non-standard treatments. While I have seen every type of treatment have efficacy, I noted that some may work for some patients and not be helpful for others. A successful treatment for a man with a low grade cancer may be useless when a new and different high grade tumor begins separate from the original and controlled disease. We are also learning that the bacteria in the stomach and intestines vary widely in people. This affects the way oral medications are absorbed by the body. The same is true of the acidity balances in the stomach and small intestine. There are ways to re-establish the normal values in the gastrointestinal tract and the reader is advised to investigate this area if oral preparations are not working as expected.

A gentleman from Virginia was seeing me every three months to evaluate his tumor. Four times a year he would try a different alternative treatment. I would confirm the beneficial effect for him on each of his visits. On a subsequent appointment I noted a high grade vascular prostate tumor that started invading his bladder on the left side. He went overseas for intense herbal and immune system treatments. Upon his quarterly return, the left side was inactive but the right side of the prostate gland with low grade cancer had now become aggressive and invaded the right side of the bladder. Finally, he found a regimen that controlled his tumors for the time being. My patients have taught me much and I acknowledge them for their courage in self healing. As long as I can continue to keep an open mind, I will be able to effectively explore, develop, refine and share new healing modalities.

The approach I advocate for decision-making about prostate cancer detection, diagnosis and treatment is based on 39 years experience in the field of diagnostic ultrasound, 20 years of imaging the prostate with power Doppler blood flows and 10 years of performing 3-D power Doppler sonograms (3D PDS); it is also based on comparing my results with high resolution MRI scans of the pelvis with special sequences formulated specifically for the prostate. I have diagnosed, observed and shared in the treatment of some 7,900 patients. Two men have died from their prostate cancer in this last 10-year period. One young man, 42 years old, could not be saved by any type of conventional or unconventional treatment due to the virulent malignancy that raced uncontrolled through his body despite all efforts. Another 69-year old corporate executive was in such disbelief that for 11 months after my diagnosis he denied he had highly aggressive cancer. He flew in from Los Angeles twice a year for four years until I felt a nodule and showed him a new tumor. He refused to accept this was a cancer and each month he would call me and ask, "Could it be an infection? Could it be from an old injury? Could my weekly prostate massage have caused this? What about my foreign travel exposures? Could riding my bicycle on very bumpy roadways produce this?" After a year of questions, to which I could only reply, "It is possible, but I strongly advise immediate biopsy and definitive treatment," the malignancy finally blocked his bladder and he could no longer urinate, which is a very late sign of widespread cancer. When a biopsy was performed, it showed a Gleason 5+4 (highly malignant), and sadly he succumbed a year later.

Besides personal experience, my evaluations and recommendations are based on seeking out practical knowledge in the field of medicine. In 1972, I asked my colleague, Dr. Smith, the senior ultrasound physician at Harvard Medical School, where he had trained in the fledgling field of diagnostic ultrasound. He referred me to Dr. Hans Holm, Professor of Urology at the Gentofte Hospital outside of Copenhagen, Denmark. I left New York and went to study with Dr. Holm and his staff. Not only did I learn more about sonography, I also experienced aspects of medicine that were unfathomable by American standards. For instance, kidney, liver and pancreatic tumors were being localized, and biopsies were taken with ultrasound guidance. American surgeons were taught at that time (and are still cautioned today) that biopsies of the pancreas are to be avoided if possible because puncturing the pancreas will leak deadly digestive enzymes producing life threatening peritonitis (inflammation of the lining of the abdominal cavity). During my first week at this Danish teaching hospital and medical center I saw many biopsies of the kidneys and liver without complications. At the end of that week, a Danish fisherman required a pancreatic biopsy for a mass located in the upper abdomen. Dr. Holm numbed the skin of the abdomen, put an 8 inch long needle into the pancreas under ultrasound guidance while the locally anesthetized patient was still awake and removed a core of tissue. Then, the lower level surgeons repeated the procedure, as did the Danish medical residents in training and finally myself. On morning rounds at 7:00 a.m. the next day, the patient—who had no less than 32 biopsies of his pancreas—was complaining that he didn't like the clear liquid breakfast he was served. He wanted real food!

Twenty two years ago my father, then a practicing physician, had one of the first PSA tests. It registered 14, very much above the 4 ng/ml level considered normal, and strongly indicated cancer. My sonogram on his prostate showed nothing suspicious. He never had a PSA exam again and never developed clinical prostate cancer. I had a PSA test 15 years ago as part of a routine physical. It measured 22 ng/ml. This was 550% above the normal value! I had just started performing power

Doppler sonograms and did one on myself. There was no abnormality. I now refuse to have the PSA exam performed on myself. Twelve years ago the Director of the National Cancer Institute of Australia refused to endorse PSA tests. He publicly stated that the cure was worse than the disease. He kept his personal prostate philosophy and lost his job. In the greater New York City area, most physicians politely decline PSA blood tests on themselves.

Not only do some insurance companies decline to accept a man for coverage with an elevated score, but some physicians treat an abnormal number with antibiotics hoping to lower the reading that may be due to inflammation. This practice has the unfortunate effect of creating bacterial resistance to generally effective antibiotics, creating treatment difficulties when true bacterial prostate infection occurs.

When I attended the major radiology conference in Europe in Paris, called *Journees Francaises Radiologie* (JFR 2003) in October 2003, I used the 3-D technology for imaging the prostate that also gave holographic reconstructions of the capsule and vasculature of the gland. I had brought patients with me who had biopsy-proven tumors that I tested on the newer European and Japanese ultrasound units not yet available in the United States. I chose a European designed unit that had a specific probe for dedicated prostate scanning. Although the probe was in clinical use all over the world and even approved by the FDA in the US, there was not one being used in North America for prostate cancer diagnosis. As of this writing, according to the manufacturer, I am one of the few physicians using the European-designed Kretz ultrahigh resolution automated 3-D power Doppler system in the Americas for prostate diagnosis and treatment follow up, and the reason is because urologists use the sonogram primarily to guide the prostate needle biopsy. On the other hand, radiologists do not see patients for this type of exam, since urologists tend not to refer their patients to radiologists. Nor do patients ask for a radiologist when they have prostate problems. My goal has been to inform patients about advanced international medical diagnostic modalities and offer new treatment options. This led me to change my profession from diagnostic radiologist to interventional radiologist, where I tailor treatment to the patient based on newer concepts in radiologic imaging as I maintain sensitivity to the patient's lifestyle choices regarding therapy. I have been inspired by my patients to do more than give diagnoses and recommend possible treatment choices. I work with the patient's team of urologist, internist, chemotherapist and radiotherapist to assure seamless integration of therapeutic suggestions. I now also search for and bring back newer therapies, and practice them in the US if FDA approved (and out of the US if not FDA approved). Through my patients' generous financial support to the Biofoundation for Angiogenesis Research and Development, I am able to discover, evaluate and incorporate better treatment protocols into my practice.

In my earlier book, I suggested that lasers could be used to treat cancers in a focal manner. This wish has come to pass and uses MRI and 3D PDS to accurately insert a laser fiber directly into a tumor and destroy it in about 6 minutes. Since this is done under local anesthesia sparing the patient the cost and side effects of general anesthesia, I have asked Dr. Dan Sperling, the inventor of this treatment to add the following chapter. This treatment so far has no side effects although it has been in use for two years worldwide. While we don't yet have published cancer control data on this therapy (as of this writing) we anticipate that it will compare favorably with the 10-30% recurrence of tumor following HIFU (High Intensity Focused Ultrasound) therapy and most radiation therapies. Time will tell if this extraordinary technology will replace many other standard treatments; however, the treatment includes destroying an extra margin of tissue around the cancer for added insurance that the cancer has been eradicated by the laser. The treatment continues until this has been achieved and documented by the 3D PDS (power Doppler) and DCE (contrast) MRI, thereby adding confidence as to its efficacy. This treatment uses the transrectal approach as does HIFU and the only reported complication so far was a man complaining that his hemorrhoids were bleeding. By contrast, with HIFU we have seen urethral strictures with difficulty urinating as a common side effect shortly after the catheter has been removed.

CHAPTER 6

FOCAL LASER ABLATION OF PROSTATE TUMORS

By Dan Sperling, MD

One looks back with appreciation to the brilliant teachers,
but with gratitude to those who touched our human feelings.
—Carl Jung

Before I tackle the content of this chapter, I want to express my appreciation and gratitude to Dr. Robert Bard, who invited me to contribute a chapter to this unique and valuable book. For 40 years, Dr. Bard has dedicated his work to researching the field of prostate cancer, including the nature of the disease and effective treatments. There is no question that he is an authority on his chosen subject, and an expert at imaging. Just as important, he understands with his mind and his heart the patient's world, and the desire for curative treatments that preserve and enhance quality of life. His compassion touches the human feelings of countless patients. It is an honor to be asked to contribute a chapter to his fine book.

Dr. Bard and I share a passion to contribute to the evolution of prostate cancer care. While I am fortunate that there has been no prostate cancer in my immediate family, I have known men who have suffered from this disease. I have also known men who suffered as a result of treating it. A tragic example is a friend's father who had his prostate removed. To this day, he wears diapers and lacks erectile function. Like Dr. Bard, I knew there had to be a better treatment.

Historically, prostate cancer has been the province of urologists. In my own career as a radiologist, my gateway into the world of prostate cancer was imaging. My interest was sparked during my Residency, and expanded during my Fellowship in Body and Internal Imaging. My main focus was on cancer (oncologic) imaging. I was initially enthusiastic about PET scans (Positron Emission Tomography is an imaging test that uses a radioactive substance called a tracer to look for disease in the body) because they were fantastic for most types of organ cancers. However, they were disappointingly inadequate for prostate tumors. My frustration grew as patients were sent for PET scans or CT scans (Computerized Tomography is a technology that combines a series of X-ray views taken from many different angles and computer processing to create cross-sectional images) which offered a high level of detection except for prostate cancer. Back then, MRI (Magnetic Resonance Imaging uses a harmless magnetic field in combination with radio waves to generate pictures of structures inside the body) was not yet where it is today. I knew I had to wait for imaging technology to become more advanced.

As I pursued ongoing clinical education, attended conferences and read journal articles, a few articles from a Dutch group caught my attention. I learned that radiologists at the University Medical Center in Nijmegen (pronounced NYE-mi-gan) in The Netherlands were using MRI to guide prostate biopsies. I immediately grasped the potential for precision targeting of biopsy needles because conventional ultrasound as used by urologists in their offices could not give the visual clarity of MRI. I decided to pursue training in Nijmegen with Drs. Jurgen Futterer and Jelle Barentsz, and headed to Europe.

I quickly developed a solid professional relationship with Jurgen Futterer. By the time I had returned to the U.S. I had decided that he would be an incredible person with whom I could collaborate as I explored ways to improve prostate tumor detection and diagnosis. Intuitively, I knew that this would contribute not only to medical science, but also to quality of life for men whose rising PSA triggers a rush to an invasive and often inaccurate prostate biopsy. Just as Dr. Bard advanced detection through his work with 3D PDS ultrasound, and diagnosis by pinpointing tumor blood flow, those of us who understand the power of sophisticated imaging are shaping the future of prostate cancer medicine.

Eventually, Dr. Futterer came to the U.S. so we could identify how MRI could be utilized in the prostate. At the same time, more powerful MRI equipment was becoming available. One reason why my early experience with MRI fell short of my expectations was the low strength of earlier machines. The greater the strength, the better the images. Here's a good explanation from "How Stuff Works"[4]:

> The biggest and most important component in an MRI system is the magnet. The magnet in an MRI system is rated using a unit of measure known as a Tesla. Another unit of measure commonly used with magnets is the gauss (1 Tesla = 10,000 gauss). The magnets in use today in MRI are in the 0.5-Tesla to 3.0-Tesla range, or 5,000 to 30,000 gauss. Extremely powerful magnets—up to 60 Tesla—are used in research. Compared with the earth's 0.5-gauss magnetic field, you can see how incredibly powerful these magnets are.

It is common to shorten the word Tesla simply to the letter T. At the time of my early training, almost all diagnostic MRI scans were done using 1.5 T magnets. Remember that these are very expensive pieces of equipment, so as 2T magnets became available, an imaging center would likely look carefully at its budget before replacing an earlier model with an updated machine. However, my desire remained: to gain access to the best available magnet. My teamwork with Dr. Futterer reinforced my commitment. Today, I am fortunate to have access to a 3T magnet, thus producing excellent prostate images.

There is one more aspect of imaging the prostate, and that has to do with the software I use for amplifying, clarifying and analyzing the MRI images along several different lines. It uses a comprehensive set of advanced visualization tools for performing real-time image analysis of prostate MRI studies. By adjusting the prostate images using various parameters (called **multiparametric MRI**) I am able to interpret specific types of tissue with tremendous accuracy. I can clearly detect "regions of interest" (areas suspicious for tumors) and identify their size, shape, and location. From there, I can formulate a hypothesis of which areas are "clinically

4   http://www.howstuffworks.com/question698.htm

significant" (likely to be aggressive) and therefore indicate a need for a targeted MRI-guided biopsy taking only a very limited numbers of needle samples; whereas other areas may be so small as to simply warrant surveillance by means of periodic MRI imaging. As Dr. Bard has already demonstrated, detection through imaging can avoid panic and a rush to over-treatment when, in many cases, patients can safely defer getting treated, or may be candidates for a focal treatment.

"Radical" vs. "focal" prostate treatment

Until the turn of the millennium, men with prostate cancer had three basic choices: surgical removal (prostatectomy), some form of radiation treatment (external beam radiation or radioactive seed implants) or watchful waiting (with or without lifestyle management of the cancer, usually called Active Surveillance). If they opted for treatment, in most cases the treatment they received was a **radical treatment,** meaning the intent was to remove or destroy the **entire gland,** healthy or not, leaving the prostate gone or nonfunctional.

- Surgical removal (prostatectomy) is *radical* treatment because the entire gland is removed. If the tumor has penetrated the capsule, the surgeon may also take one or both neurovascular bundles (that control erection) and/or the seminal vesicles.
- Radiation therapy was also a *radical* treatment in the sense that the whole gland was radiated. However, radiation effects are not immediate, but rather gradual and cumulative as it damages the cells' internal ability to reproduce. If cancer returns, there is often a buildup of complicated scarring that makes surgical removal difficult. In addition, the tumor may be more aggressive than the original tumor, because the hardier cells were able to survive, or even mutate into a more dangerous line of cancer.

Radical treatments carry the risk of urinary, sexual and bowel side effects. The walnut-sized prostate is so important that Mother Nature has made access difficult, and surrounded it closely with other vital structures that are hard to avoid when a surgeon goes in with a scalpel, or radiation scatters.

Despite the risk of side effects, treating the whole gland was considered essential. Doctors were taught that prostate cancer is a **multifocal disease**, meaning that if cancer cells were found in one place in the gland, there must be other cells lurking throughout the gland, even if only microscopic. It was therefore assumed that the only safe way to treat prostate cancer was to obliterate the whole source, so there could be no chance of future growth or of the cancer coming back. The problem was, and continues to be, that radical treatments are NOT 100% guaranteed! This needs a little explaining. Historically, before the era of PSA blood screening that began in the mid-1980s, many prostate cancers were discovered only when they were quite advanced. Early stage prostate cancer rarely makes itself known because there are few, if any, symptoms. Prior to the PSA blood test, many patients suspected nothing until urination became difficult, or there was blood in their urine, or they began experiencing back or hip pain. Remember: there were no imaging technologies that could identify tumors within the gland, and the digital rectal exam (DRE) cannot identify more than a limited range of tumor activity. Sadly, many patients who were diagnosed and treated with surgery or radiation may already have had cancer that had spread, or metastasized, outside of the prostate capsule. Not only was their disease beyond control, an untold number of these patients suffered permanent consequences in their quality of life. Urinary leakage requiring pads or diapers, erectile dysfunction, and bowel problems were inconvenient at best, downright humiliating at worst.

Radical treatments are still the standard of care. But let's examine an area in which radical care was first questioned, then eventually transformed: breast cancer therapies.

There are great similarities between breast cancer and prostate cancer. A nearly equivalent number of new cases are diagnosed each year (upwards of 220,000); about 1 in 6 men are expected to develop prostate cancer, and about 1 in 8 women breast cancer; both appear to be hormonally fueled, even if environmentally or genetically caused; both were originally thought to require radical treatment in order to achieve cancer control. Radical mastectomy (breast removal accompanied by removal of lymph nodes and the underlying chest muscle) was not only disfiguring, it was curiously ineffective in many cases where the breast surgeon was confident that all of the cancer was removed. Were it not for the courage of a few pioneering breast surgeons, and a larger number of daring patients for whom the consequences of radical treatment were unacceptable, the concept of a lumpectomy (just removing the localized tumor, often followed by a precautionary course of radiation and/or chemotherapy) would not be with us today.

Similarly, a small but growing number of urologists, oncologists, and interventional radiologists (those who use image guidance to penetrate the body for biopsy or treatment) have begun offering the equivalent of a focal prostate treatment, or "male lumpectomy," a term attributed to Dr. Gary Onik, an interventional radiologist. Dr. Onik examined published data showing that prostate cancer is not always multifocal. He, like myself and others, rightly asked: If we could be reasonably certain that this patient has only one clinically significant tumor, is there a minimally invasive way we can destroy the tumor? And if so, can we avoid creating urinary, sexual or bowel damage? This is the idea behind focal treatment, and this is the way to transform the world of prostate cancer therapy.

Here's how it came to me. As I was doing more MRI-guided biopsies, and becoming proficient and confident in "seeing," accessing and diagnosing prostate tumors, I attended a professional conference where I saw laser being used for skin conditions. Immediately, the precision and power of using heat generated by focused light energy struck me. I asked myself, "Can I find a way to use this localization of treatment in the prostate?"

With that question in the back of my mind, I attended an interventional conference where papers were being presented on tumor ablation (destruction) in organs like the liver, kidney, lung and breast. The presenters discussed various ablation technologies. Dr. Bard has already discussed the most common, among them being radiofrequency ablation (RF or RFA), cryotherapy (freezing) and high intensity focused ultrasound (HIFU). The problem with many of these techniques had to do with whether or not one could actually "see" the destruction occur in real time, and quickly verify the complete treatment coverage following treatment. In other words, the superior imaging offered by MRI was not necessarily practical, as it might be difficult to actually do the procedure in the bore (tube or tunnel) of the MRI equipment. Plus, urologists were not trained on MRI, nor did they generally have access to the equipment. A further difficulty with HIFU was the lack of FDA clearance to offer it in the U.S. where it has been undergoing clinical trials. Patients who didn't qualify to participate in a trial would have to pay for the treatment (not covered by Medicare or insurance) PLUS travel outside of the U.S. to have the treatment.

Nonetheless, I now had all the "dots"—all I had to do was connect them! So I approached one particular manufacturer of clinical lasers, a company called Visualase, with an idea for getting a laser fiber into a prostate tumor, using MRI guidance and a specific applicator similar to a hollow biopsy needle. They were very interested, and excited to get started. Although they had already developed a way to approach brain tumors, and were having success with it, what I brought to their work was a specific localization technology with which I was already experienced, thanks to my work with Dr. Futterer and MRI-guided prostate biopsies.

> *"The time has come," the walrus said, "to talk of many things…"*
> —**Lewis Carroll**, Through the Looking Glass

The time is ripe for focal prostate treatment because the prostate cancer world is changing. For example, what's to become of routine PSA screening? In October 2011 a U.S. Government Panel recommended discontinuing this practice for otherwise healthy men with no family history of prostate cancer. The panel's rationale partly sprang from two large-scale research studies suggesting that there is no significant survival advantage to regular blood tests. The panel was also motivated by another concern. It has long been observed that men with a rising PSA are rushed into invasive, sight-blind needle biopsies that entail risks of infection, false negatives, and under-staging. A positive biopsy triggers an intense period of decision-making with whole-gland treatment often being the physician's first recommendation.

Other groups have a very different say in the matter. If you ask patient support groups, organizations, and most urologists, you are likely to find opinion in favor of continuing routine screening. After all, aside from rising PSA (which Dr. Bard has pointed out is a flawed tool at best), early stage prostate cancer has virtually no symptoms. From this viewpoint, leaving cancer undetected might mean missing a critical window for treating it—so by the time there are symptoms it's often too late for a local treatment because "the horse is out of the barn." They argue that the intent to spare men from having unpleasant biopsies (with their risks of false negatives, nerve damage, infection, and the theory of spreading cancer via the needle tracks) and being rushed into radical treatments (with their potential urinary and sexual side effects) may be sacrificing the lives of men whose cancer is found at an advanced stage.

So here's the national dilemma around PSA screening:

1. Don't go looking for prostate cancer in the general population, as it may lead to over-treatment (Translation: trust that prostate cancer is mostly slow growing).

2. Don't wait too long to detect prostate cancer, and don't undertreat by doing anything less than a whole-gland modality (Translation: no prostate cancer can be trusted).

With this kind of ambivalence, I'm proposing a rational middle ground: focal laser ablation.

Focal Laser Ablation (FLA)

Targeted prostate cancer treatments have been performed for over a decade, most commonly by cryotherapy (freezing) and HIFU (High Intensity Focused Ultrasound). With increasing published data on focal treatment by Onik, Bahn, Ahmed and others, confidence in patient selection and follow-up mechanisms is blossoming.

A promising new modality has been added to the arsenal used to eradicate tumors. MRI-guided Focal Laser Ablation (FLA) was originally developed to treat brain tumors, and has gained broad FDA approval to treat targets in soft tissue. Thus, it is being explored not only for brain, spine and prostate lesions, but also kidney and liver tumors.

Prostate FLA should not be confused with laser-based vaporization treatments for urethral constriction due to benign prostatic enlargement, such as Green Light Laser. Prostate FLA is directed against malignancy. It uses light energy delivered by a small hollow fiber (similar to the fiber optics used in fountain-shaped novelty lamps, where a tiny glow of bright light appears at the end of each fiber). For treatment purposes, the laser fiber is threaded into a long needle-like hollow applicator, which is placed directly in the prostate under MRI imaging until the very tip is placed at the core of the tumor. No surgery is necessary, since the applicator is slender and very sharp at the open tip. As the laser fiber delivers light at the tip, temperatures in the target area begin to rise and form a globe of intense heat that destroys the tumor and an accompanying margin of safety. The area of thermal change can be observed using special imaging, so the physician can be sure of a complete and accurate treatment.

Magnetic Resonance Imaging plays a key role in FLA, and the more powerful the magnet, the more precise, responsible and reliable the ablation. Until more powerful magnets become available, it is crucial that a 3T magnet be used because it is simply faster and clearer in detail. Not only does MRI guide the treatment planning and applicator placement, the magnet is also sensitive to temperature changes in the tissue. This allows the physician to monitor and control how much energy is delivered. The procedure averages around two hours, and is done under a local prostate nerve block.

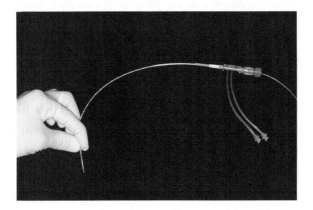

Fig 6.1 The thin (1.6mm) Visualase laser fiber is placed into the tumor under MRI guidance using minimally invasive techniques

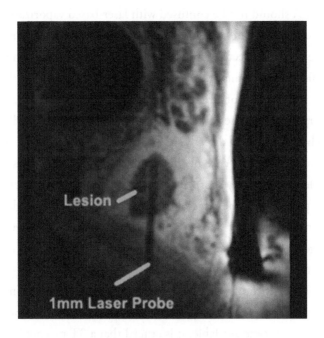

Fig 6.2 Pre-procedure MRI confirms
placement of applicator in the target tissue

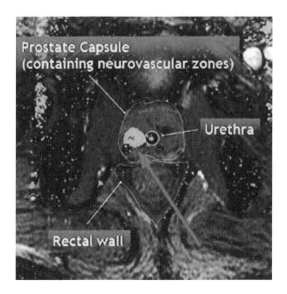

Fig 6.3 The laser is activated to begin heating of the tumor. Using MR images and Visualase software allows the physician to see the tissue heating during laser irradiation, and control how much energy is delivered

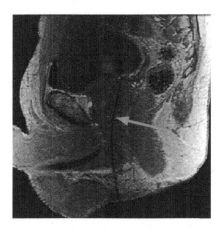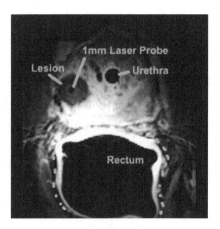

Fig 6.4 and 6.5 Results are confirmed with MR images. The laser applicator is removed and the small incision is closed with one stitch and/or a bandage. The entire procedure lasts approximately 1.5 to 3 hours, and often requires only mild conscious sedation or even just local anesthetic. Patient often returns home the same day with no catheter[5]

---

5   Images courtesy of Visualase, Inc. and available at www.visualaseinc.com

Advantages of focal laser ablation include: local anesthesia; MRI guidance under a 3T magnet; rapid recovery, usually same day; and no catheter. Most importantly, of the 70+ patients I have treated, all have preserved urinary and sexual function because of how precise the laser is.

Conditions for focal treatment

Recent evidence from prostate cancer pathology studies of surgically removed prostate glands suggests that not all prostate tumors are multifocal.[6] Furthermore, as new imaging technologies such as Dr. Bard's 3D PDS or my 3T MRI and specialized software allow superior differentiation of tissue within the gland over conventional gray scale ultrasound, the ability to target biopsy needles into areas of interest results in "… better characterization of the biopsy-proven cancer, to determine the higher-grade and greater-volume cancers as 'important,' as well as the lower-grade and smaller-volume cancers as 'indolent.'"[7] In other words, prostate malignancy is not necessarily multifocal, and with advanced imaging many tumors can be identified when they are early stage, low-risk, and small in size. Furthermore, there is an increasing body of research and a growing number of specialty conferences dedicated to focal ablation. International experts are in dialogue to identify reasonable conditions for focal therapy. Criteria under consideration include: number of disease foci (more than one focus of disease); size of index (primary or largest) lesion if more than one foci exist; tumor location; biopsy-demonstrated Gleason grade of all disease foci; psychological appropriateness of patient; informed consent; and patient commitment to follow-up protocol. Consensus is evolving on what constitutes clinically significant vs. clinically insignificant disease, that is, tumors that warrant treatment vs. those that are amenable to Active Surveillance, focal ablation, and monitoring through imaging and biological serum markers.

My dual rationale for laser ablation

My first rationale for FLA comes from professional journals and conferences. From a clinical perspective, as I follow the literature and attend conferences on focal treatment of prostate cancer, I am convinced that the data is compelling and justifies this approach for properly qualified patients. Multiparametric MRI

---

6   Iczkowski KA, Hossain D, Torklo KC, Qian J, Jucia MS, Wheeler TM, Rewcastle JC, Bostwick DG, Department of Pathology, University of Colorado Health Science Center, Denver, CO. Preoperative prediction of unifocal, unilateral, margin-negative, and small volume prostate cancer. Urologic Oncol: Seminars and Original Investigations 2008 Nov;26(2): 681-82.

7   Ukimura O, Faber K, Gill IS. Intra-prostatic targeting. Curr Opin Urol 2012 Mar;22(2):97-103.

allows clear definition of tumors as small as 4 mm. For FLA, I can place the laser probe into the core of the tumor, and ablate (destroy) a zone that includes an encompassing margin of safety. In addition, I require a diligent two-year follow up program of quarterly multiparametric imaging under a 3T magnet, and a targeted biopsy into the ablation zone at six months.

For my other rationale, I turn to the world of patients. They talk to me about the "trifecta" they are looking for: success in the bedroom, bathroom and cancer control. To date, I am happy that my patients experience the first two successes. I am expecting the laser to deliver equivalent cancer control with other focal modalities. For example, a recent prospective study out of the Urology Department of University College London demonstrated 92% freedom from clinically significant PCa after treatment with focal HIFU[8] which also uses extreme heat, though created by sound energy rather than light energy. It goes without saying that, just as with other current focal modalities, should cancer recur in the non-treated tissue, no treatment bridges have been burned. In such cases, patients would have the choice of any treatment option from radical to focal that is appropriate for the stage and grade of recurrence.

As clinical ambivalence over PSA testing filters into the patient world, here are some of the questions men and their loved ones struggle with:

1. Should I have an annual PSA blood test?
2. Should I rush to have a biopsy based on an elevated PSA?
3. Isn't a TRUS biopsy "blind" to tissue differences, and will it miss a small tumor altogether?
4. If one or more needles contain cancer, how can I be sure the level of aggression has been reliably identified?
5. My doctor recommends not waiting too long to get treated. Can I trust him/her to tell me the truth about the side effects of radical treatment?
6. If I want to hold off on treatment, how can I be sure I'm a candidate for Active Surveillance?
7. If I hold off on treatment, is PSA sensitive enough to monitor tumor growth?
8. My doctor thinks I'm a candidate for focal treatment. How can I be sure I really am?

---

8   Ahmed HU, Hindley RD, Dickinson L, Freeman A, Kirkham AP, Sahu M., Scott R, Allen C, Van der Meulen J, Emberton M. Focal therapy for localized unifocal and multifocal prostate cancer: a prospective development study. Lancet Oncol 2012 Jun; 13(6):622-32.

Just as the advent of image-guided targeted biopsy brings an accurate, minimalist, effective alternative to 12+ core TRUS biopsies, Focal Laser Ablation brings an accurate, minimalist, effective alternative to either doing nothing, or doing too much. FLA may not be the "silver bullet" patients are wishing for, but for those with demonstrated focal disease verified by advanced imaging, it resolves today's dilemma between too much treatment vs. delaying treatment. It also interfaces beautifully with the kind of lifestyle changes, which I wholeheartedly endorse, that may reduce the possibility of recurrence by altering the genes that regulate tumor growth, as demonstrated by a recent study conducted by Dean Ornish, MD.[9] For all these reasons, FLA contributes to the evolution of prostate cancer treatment.

When patients come to me, they're looking to maintain their quality of life. Men are living longer, maintaining active lives with high quality. When diagnosed with prostate cancer and faced with treatment, they're worried about their dignity, their self-esteem, their love life. And of course, everyone's concerned with spread and death.

Not everyone is a candidate for FLA. Even for men who are, a certain percentage will psychologically be more comfortable with surgery or other whole gland treatment. They strongly feel, "I can't live with the idea that my cancer might still there." I encourage them to speak to multiple specialists and get their opinion. It's a personal decision. There are patients for whom potency is not an issue, and radical treatment will be a good choice for them.

For those men who are clinically qualified for focal treatment, and who are comfortable with leaving behind a living, functional prostate gland because they know it can be monitored by imaging, focal laser ablation is an elegant, minimalist treatment with maximum preservation of lifestyle. As Dr. Bard and I both recognize, new imaging has opened new pathways to prostate tumor treatment.

---

9   Ornish, D. Changing your lifestyle can change your genes, Prostate Cancer Communication, Jun 2011, 19-20.

CHAPTER 7

ASSESSING TREATMENT RESPONSE

Standard medical practice suggests that the following are useful guides for evaluating the cancer's response to therapy, in this case prostate cancer:

a. Clinical exam

b. Imaging–CT, MRI, 3D PDS, isotope scans, PET/CT

c. Tumor markers–PSA

d. Performance status

e. Sexual function

f. Urinary function

g. Quality of life

h. Survival

The value of medical imaging is to:

- Determine efficacy of therapy
- Monitor changes

- Tailor future therapy
- Determine tumor recurrence
- Identify new tumor

Imaging after treatment

One of the problems of evaluating cancer treatment is that the tumor may be rendered harmless or even dead but the volume of the tumor remains the same. That is, the cancer cells may be killed off and scar tissue replaces the dead cells, leaving the size of the original malignancy unchanged. This lesson was learned 15 years ago in treating liver tumors. The therapy would render the cancer harmless, but the size of the mass on the isotope scans, sonogram, CT and MRI would remain unchanged or even enlarge. The same is true of some prostate cancers that are inactivated but still feel like cancer on the digital rectal exam and show a mass effect on the sonogram and MRI. There needs to be a way to monitor changes and determine the efficacy of treatment. A common medical solution to this dilemma has been to obtain multiple needle biopsies some interval after the procedure and look for cancer cells under the microscope.

3D PDS after treatment

Fortunately, the blood flows in malignancies that have been inactivated decrease or disappear and can be quickly and accurately measured in the moment. Thus, with 3D PDS there is a simple tool to quantify blood flow patterns to demonstrate therapeutic response. In fact, combining 3D PDS with contrast enhanced MRI has major clinical potential. We have found dramatic blood flow reductions in tumors within minutes of treatment with thermal ablations. This visual confirmation provides substantial relief to the patient and often precludes the need for multiple biopsies. Dr. Bruno Fornage's 2005 study, published in *American Journal of Radiology*, showed that the blood flow in vascular tumors disappeared completely after fifteen minutes of radiofrequency ablation providing an exact endpoint of the therapy. RFA is particularly useful in embolizing (blocking tumor blood vessels) vascular prostate disorders and the effect shows immediately. If vessels were not fully blocked, the procedure can be repeated within minutes. The pathologist can see if the tumor has died and scarred down or turned into a benign jelly; however, the microscope cannot always confirm that intact appearing cancers are inactivated and essentially harmless or possibly remain virulent and life threatening.

PET scan after treatment

PET or Positron Emission Tomography, a nuclear isotope diagnostic tool has not been used much for evaluation of the prostate in the United States. A grant from the U.S. Department of Energy and the National Institute of Health to Japanese investigators Drs. Oyama and Akino showed new modifications may prove clinically useful. This work was presented at the 2005 AUA Meeting. Likewise, a German study presented at the same meeting by Dr. Uwe Teiber showed PET was useful in detecting lymph node metastases better than CT scans and recommended further studies using the combination of PET/CT scanners. Yet another German group of urologists, Dr. Machtens and others, developed evidence that nuclear isotope scans with new generation radioactive tracers looked promising for the future as a prostate cancer detection tool. The physicians from the European cancer center in Ulm, Germany showed yet another nuclear isotope was useful in detecting local cancer recurrence. Dr. Bartsch concluded, "...PET/CT is a promising diagnostic tool...able to demonstrate local lesions responsible for rising PSA...which could be verified by aimed transrectal ultrasound guided biopsy." In another paper at the AUA 2005 by Dr. Bartsch and colleagues, he reported 95% accuracy in detecting metastatic lymph nodes with PET/CT scans compared with operative findings. A paper by American radiologist in Texas, Dr. Joseph Basler and associates, following Dr. Bartsch's talk, showed that a Veterans Administration study of the lymph node drainage of the prostate demonstrated a different path than expected. This presentation funded by the University of Texas Health Sciences Center cautioned "...the current method of obturator node dissection with radical prostatectomy is inadequate and may explain a proportion of patients who fail local treatment despite adequate margin and traditional negative node status." A Swiss paper by Dr. D. Schmid, presented in 2005 *Radiology*, recommended PET/CT for detecting local cancer recurrence and lymph node metastases. He recommended this test since MR detection of lymph node metastases had a low sensitivity and it has been shown that lymph node size does not correlate with the presence of prostate cancer metastases.

MRI imaging after treatment

New MRI protocols to improve lymph node detection have been developed in the Netherlands by Dr. Jelle Barentsz, radiologist and President of the International Cancer Imaging Society. Pelvic lymph node metastases have a significant impact on the prognosis of patients with prostate cancer. Small lymph nodes involved with tumor spread means local treatments such as surgery and HIFU are not curative. Surgical lymph node detection has usually been performed by operative dissection of the pelvis. This was necessary since CT and MRI use size criteria to determine the presence or absence of disease. This means that nodes larger than 7 mm are suspicious but not definitive and may be due to inflammation or other non cancerous entities. Unfortunately, the prostate cancer tends to produce small areas called micrometastases that are often smaller than 7 mm and sometimes as tiny as 3 mm. A new MRI technique (LNMRI or Lymph Node MRI) using harmless iron oxide (rust) particles has shown to be 90% specific in predicting metastases and 98% specific in determining that there are no malignant areas. This requires a standard MRI and injection one day prior to the special MRI to re-image and observe abnormal lymph node areas. The test can detect tumor foci as small as 3 mm. A map of the malignant nodes is obtained which may be used for intensity modulated radiotherapy (IMRT) or other treatments. Diseased areas may be given more radiation and unaffected areas spared treatment. This work was presented at the 2008 *International Radiology Society* meeting. According to Dr. Jurgen Futterer, co-author of *Image Guided Prostate Cancer Treatments* (Springer 2013), newer lymph node imaging technologies are being studied in Europe and may be applicable to the prostate in the near future.

What is the role of the Prostate Specific Antigen (PSA) in this scenario? Some men who have had their prostates removed surgically still have measurable PSA levels. It is thought that this is most likely due to recurrent tumor formation in the post-op site, although many times no cancer is ever found. Researchers from Memorial Sloan Kettering Cancer Center have found that the levels of PSA fluctuate normally and have recommended a repeat blood test if a post-op elevation occurred. In this scenario, sophisticated imaging done by an expert reader would be a preferable diagnostic indicator as to whether or not treatment had been a success.

CHAPTER 8

REFLECTIONS ON CONVENTIONAL TREATMENTS

The times they are a-changin'.
—Bob Dylan

xciting and imaginative medical technologies in the world of cancer detection, diagnosis and treatment are always in progress. Both informed decision making (IDM) and shared decision making (SDM) rest on a foundation of full disclosure so physician and patient alike have access to all options available at that time. One aspect of that information includes knowledge of ongoing clinical trials that can be easily found on the internet at www.clinicaltrials.gov. There, patients may learn that they qualify to be part of an investigational study of an experimental imaging or treatment modality that they can only access through that study.

The primary purpose of this book is to acquaint patients with information that they may not get from their own doctors—for any number of reasons, so no finger-pointing implied! However, the content of this book would be incomplete without briefly reflecting on some conventional (standard) prostate cancer treatments. After all, the times may indeed be a-changin', but thousands of empowered, informed patients will continue to choose surgery (radical prostatectomy), radiation, cryotherapy, and (for advanced or metastatic prostate cancer) ADT (androgen deprivation therapy). Although countless books and internet articles go far more deeply into these topics, here are some things to think about when considering each of them.

With so many promising innovations, why prostatectomy?

Following are important points regarding prostatectomy for both patients and physicians alike to keep in mind:

- It is the only option that removes the entire prostate, whereas other options leave viable tissue and possible cancer behind.
- Surgery is the only option that provides accurate staging, volume, tumor, grade, and margins.
- Rates of both upgrading (higher Gleason grade found on the final pathology than on biopsy) and upstaging (higher pathological stage than initial clinical stage) are approximately 30% each after prostatectomy; the true pathology would be otherwise unknown with either radiotherapy or ablation.
- Follow-up is straightforward. PSA should be undetectable following a prostatectomy with negative surgical margins. PSA continues to be produced following radiation and is difficult to interpret.
- There is no risk of a secondary malignancy developing due to radiation.
- Prostatectomy provides relief of any prior or future bladder outlet obstruction due to benign prostatic hyperplasia (BPH).
- Radiation is still an option after surgery, whereas salvage prostatectomy after radiation remains a difficult and morbid operation.
- Many patients benefit psychologically from knowing that the cancer is physically removed from the body.

History

Retropubic radical prostatectomy (RRP) was first reported by Millin in 1947. The surgery was associated with significant morbidity: high blood loss often requiring transfusion, incontinence, impotence, and prolonged recovery. In the early 1980s

Walsh described a new, more precise nerve-sparing technique of anatomical dissection that improved functional outcomes. Schuessler performed the first laparoscopic radical prostatectomy (LRP) in 1991; the technique was later refined and popularized by Guilloneau and others in the late 1990s. It has since been demonstrated to be safe, effective, and similar to RRP in oncologic outcomes. LRP provided the benefits of decreased blood loss (secondary to the increased abdominal pressure of the pneumoperitoneum and better visualization) and a minimally invasive approach but remained a technically challenging operation with a steep learning curve and poor ergonomics.

Robotic-assisted laparoscopic prostatectomy (RALP) was first reported by Abbou et al in 2000. It was popularized by Menon et al as a minimally invasive technique with vastly improved ergonomics and shorter learning curve relative to LRP. In particular, RALP offered 3-dimensional stereoscopic visualization and intuitive finger-controlled movements with range of motion surpassing that of the human hand. Robotic prostatectomy is now beginning to surpass both open and laparoscopic approaches in outcomes as robotic surgeons become more proficient.

Why the robotic approach?

The robotic approach has evolved because there is still substantial room for improving important outcomes after open surgery. Urologists continue to seek ways to refine prostatectomy techniques. However, the robotic revolution is also patient-driven. Patients continue to seek out minimally invasive surgical approaches, hoping to minimize surgical trauma. Though robotic equipment is expensive, and a high surgery volume is necessary to make the purchase and maintenance of a robot cost-effective, the fact is robotic prostatectomy is now by far the dominant surgical approach to prostate cancer, and its popularity continues to rise. A learning curve of approximately 50 to 100 cases must be overcome before a level of efficiency can be obtained that will achieve financial viability. Furthermore, the importance of a dedicated, trained robotic OR team cannot be overemphasized. Steinberg et al examined the costs of overcoming the learning curves in 8 robotic prostatectomy series reported in the literature and concluded that RALP may be best suited to high volume prostatectomy centers.

Surgeons who already have advanced laparoscopic skills may have no better results with the robot. That being said, the robot provides several advantages for most surgeons: more procedural control, better vision, greater wrist flexibility, suturing facility, instrument stability, and surgeon comfort.

Whether laparoscopic or robotic-assisted laparoscopic, both approaches are considered less invasive than the traditional open prostatectomy. There are other considerations for RALP:

- Though long-term oncologic efficacy data are as yet lacking for RALP, reported positive margin rates are usually improved compared to the open approach. For example, Smith et al noted a positive margin rate of 15% compared to a rate of 35% for the open approach. It should be noted, however, that patients in their open prostatectomy series had an overall higher risk profile (higher Gleason scores, PSA values, etc.), thereby possibly confounding the data.

- A common criticism of robotic surgery is that the lack of tactile feedback inherent to using the robot compromises the surgeon's ability to judge whether cancer has breached the prostatic pseudocapsule and therefore diminishes cancer control. To counter this claim, many robotic surgeons point out that the superb visualization (11x magnification and 3-dimensional view) more than compensates for this.

- With regard to postoperative complications, incidences are mostly similar, with the exception of a very low bladder neck contracture rate with the robot (<1%).

- Many studies have reported less post-operative pain with the robotic approach.

- Blood loss is unquestionably less. This is an especially important point when dealing with patients who refuse blood transfusions, such as Jehovah's Witnesses.

- OR time has in most series been slightly longer for robotic, with more experienced robotic surgeons having shorter OR times. Our mean operative time is 127 minutes.

- Length of stay is typically less for robotic prostatectomy. Nelson et al reported a 95% rate of discharge after one hospital day vs. 82% for open surgery.

- Continence: Smith et al demonstrated a faster return to continence in 3 months, but by 12 months the difference was less marked (94% vs. 97%).

- Potency: Bilateral nerve-sparing radical prostatectomy is now the standard of care for localized disease with no evidence of extracapsular extension or frank involvement of the neurovascular bundles. Continued improvements in robotic technique, including eliminating the use of cautery during the dissection of the neurovascular bundles, have improved potency rates. Potency rates at one year are mostly in the range of 70% to 90%, though some have reported potency as high as 97%.

- Though recent articles have pointed out lower satisfaction rates and higher regret among patients who have undergone RALP compared to open prostatectomy, authors have also pointed out that these findings may be due to inappropriate expectations of the new procedure.

Radiation therapy

There are two main types of radiation therapy: external beam and brachytherapy (radioactive seed implantation). Delivery of external beam radiation continues to be refined to minimize the radiation dose to the prostate. Intensity-modulated radiation therapy (IMRT) and proton radiation therapy are essentially variations on this theme, but their availability is currently somewhat limited due to cost and/ or complexity.

With brachytherapy, radioactive seeds or needles are implanted directly into the prostate gland using ultrasound guidance to deliver a high dose of radiation to the tumor. Brachytherapy is relatively easy to perform and therefore has become popular for treatment of patients with clinically localized prostate cancer, but it is seldom used for the treatment of high-volume, high-risk prostate cancers. Urinary symptoms are more common after brachytherapy than after external beam radiotherapy, especially in patients with prostatic hyperplasia.

Both treatments result in acute symptoms of proctitis or cystitis in approximately one third of patients; 5% to 10% develop permanent disorders related to bowel, bladder, and/ or urethral function. Approximately half of patients develop erectile dysfunction, depending on age and preoperative erectile function.

Patients with a high PSA level, high Gleason score, or large-volume tumor may benefit from androgen deprivation therapy in conjunction with radiotherapy or the combination of brachytherapy and external-beam radiation. NOTE: numerous studies document increased risk of secondary bladder and rectal malignancies after radiation for prostate cancer.

Androgen deprivation therapy (ADT)

The use of androgen deprivation therapy (ADT or hormone therapy or hormone blockage) means using medication to block the production of testosterone, which appears to "feed" the growth of prostate cancer. It is successful in that it "stops cancer in its tracks" but only for some period of time before the cancer becomes "refractory" (resistant) and can no longer be controlled this way. Traditionally, ADT has been most often prescribed for advanced (metastatic) prostate cancer when local therapy is not appropriate (the cancer has already been proven to have spread beyond the capsule at time of diagnosis) or when local therapy has failed (nonlocalized recurrence after surgery, radiation, or other treatment).

However, the prescribing of ADT for localized prostate cancer ("primary ADT") has increased markedly in the last decade. An observational database of 7,195 patients with prostate cancer, including 3,439 men diagnosed since 1989, with clinical staging information available was reviewed. The data showed that patients with clinically localized prostate cancer are increasingly receiving androgen deprivation therapy before or along with radical prostatectomy, radiation therapy, or brachytherapy, although the appropriate role of hormonal therapy in localized disease is unknown. That said, primary ADT may be appropriate for older men, those with significant medical conditions precluding the use of curative therapy, or those who do not wish to undergo curative therapy. Again, it is never curative, and remissions are not infrequent.

The full impact of increased hormonal therapy use on prostate cancer mortality patterns is unknown, according to Cooperberg's article in the *Journal of the National Cancer Institute,* 2003. While there is a consensus about the use of hormone blockade, there is frequently no agreement about the type of blockade to be used or to the optimal duration of treatment. Current studies are trying to clarify this issue, but it will probably take years for this to occur. A logical approach to use for the selection and duration of the hormone treatment is to modulate the intensity of the blockade to the degree of cancer risk. This means stronger treatment for patients with more aggressive disease.

The input of the patient regarding the treatment intensity has little meaning, if the patient doesn't understand the benefits of the particular therapy or the potential side effects. Many of the possible side effects are reversible or preventable with simple measures. For example, osteoporosis (weak bones that fracture), a common side effect may be prevented with a once a week dose of Fosamax or Actonex coupled with weight training. The two other feared complications are loss of libido and energy deterioration.

Libido is a passionate attraction to the opposite sex—in other words, desire. This needs to be contrasted with potency, which is the ability to get an erection adequate for vaginal penetration. During hormone blockade, 90% of men over age 70 completely lose their sexual desire as compared with men under age 50 years who lose libido about 50% of the time. Libido returns to normal levels after therapy ceases and testosterone recovers more frequently in younger men. About 50% of men over age 70 undergoing two years of treatment never recover testosterone production, which can be supplemented with testosterone gels.

Hormone deprivation also depletes energy. It causes tiredness and weakness especially after 6 months of treatment. The degree varies with each patient and is related to loss of muscle tone and mass and may be counteracted with strength training. In severe cases progesterone (hormone) shots are helpful. The combination of listlessness and testosterone loss often leads to weight gain, however, dietary adjustments will compensate for this.

There are other side effects of medical castration. Hot flashes are a nuisance, but generally, tolerable. Breast growth occurs in more that 50 % of men on anti-androgen hormone therapy which may be treated with radiation therapy or estrogen blocking pills such as Femara. Osteoporosis accelerated bone mass loss occurs in post menopausal women with low estrogen levels and men deprived of testosterone. If left untreated, this leads to rib, spine and hip fractures (with a 50% mortality rate). These side effects may be contained by the modern bisphosphonate treatments such as Fosamax and Actonex pills. Severe cases may require intravenous infusions. Side effects of high dose bisphosphonates include joint pains; arthritis is most common in the hands and may be treated with over the counter preparations such as glucosamine, MSM and Super oxide dismutase (SOD). Standard nonsteroidal anti-inflammatory agents like Motrin and Celebrex are effective remedies.

Memory changes, according to the February, 2005, online edition of *Cancer* include problems with word finding, remembering names and reduction in verbal fluency. Visual recognition and visual memory are also affected. Emotional mood swings occur and may be diminished with common anti-depressant medications such as Zoloft or Paxil. Non cerebral problems include anemia, blood pressure elevation and liver injury. Blood is a mixture of red blood cells and serum (watery fluid). Anemia occurs when the oxygen carrying red cells are depleted resulting in weakness and shortness of breath. Hormone blockade normally drops the blood cell count by 20%, which is usually tolerable; however, 10% of men develop severe anemia. This is treatable with the hormone erythropoietin or synthetic Aranesp. Blood pressure swings occur both upward and downward and may be adjusted by standard medications. Liver irritation, detected by routine blood tests, may be caused by the commonly used antiandrogens Casodex and Flutamide. Minor injury will lead to severe liver damage if the medicine is not stopped. When the liver function returns to normal, for example, if Casodex was used, Eulexin may be substituted and vice versa.

Cryosurgery (cryotherapy)

Cryotherapy (minimally invasive treatment that freezes tumors at extremely cold temperatures) has been established as an appropriate and effective modality for recurrent, organ-confined prostate cancer after radiation, though its role as a primary modality is still controversial and rates of erectile dysfunction following treatment remain high (up to 80%). On the other hand, focal cryotherapy published by cryosurgery pioneers Gary Onik MD and Duke Bahn MD reveal high rates of cancer control (up to 95% in one study, including patients with Gleason scores as high as 7), zero incontinence, and upwards of 85% return to potency within a few months after treatment. Interestingly, research data (Bahn and others) implies that cryosurgery is more effective against high grade tumors (Gleason scores 7 and 8) than either prostatectomy or radiation. Perhaps this bodes well for thermal therapies (extreme heat or cold that destroys tumors immediately, unlike radiation) since destruction of the tumor and its blood supply occurs at the time of treatment, which can be validated at the time of treatment or shortly after by imaging.

HIFU

This is a non FDA approved technology that is minimally invasive using sonogram technology to guide a thermal ablation of the prostate. This may be used in a focal manner. Immediate complications include stricture of the urethra. Long term complications include impotence and incontinence. An initial 5 year study showed a recurrence rate of 30%, however, later studies are showing a lower rate of tumor regrowth. (NOTE: At the time of this writing, FDA approval has been applied for by two manufacturers of HIFU ablation devices; the application is under consideration by the FDA.)

CHAPTER 9

PROMISING SCIENTIFIC BREAKTHROUGHS

To get to the heart of the matter, this chapter is devoted to imparting information about advances in imaging for detection, diagnosis and treatment follow up to monitor how effective it was. In addition, this chapter includes descriptions of imaging advances not already covered, and minimally invasive treatments done using image guidance.

Breakthrough imaging described in this chapter

Contrast enhanced Doppler sonography (CEUS)

Sono-elastography

HyperSpectral Imaging (HSI)

PhotoAcoustic Imaging (PA)

3-Tesla MRI (3T MRI)

Contrast enhanced MRI (DCE-MRI)

Computer-aided full time point MRI (FTP-MRI)

Lymph node MRI (LNMRI)

New MRI blood flow technologies

PET and PET/CT isotope scans

Diffusion Weighted Imaging (DWI) of Prostate or Whole Body (simulates PET without radiation)

Breakthrough treatments described in this chapter

Pretreatment prostate size reduction

Radio Frequency Ablation and thermotherapies

(Focal Laser Ablation covered in Chapter 6)

Antiangiogenic drugs

Arterial embolization

Microwave hyperthermia

Irreversible electroporation

Dendritic cell immunotherapy

Nanoparticle therapies

Chemosensitivity testing and chemoembolization

Gene therapy/molecular biology

Photodynamic therapy

MRI-guided HIFU

Galvanotherapy (GT)

Laser assisted immunotherapy

Contrast enhanced Doppler sonography (CEUS)

The ability to better image blood vessels by injecting an enhancing agent intravenously has been used in Europe and Japan for several years. This is not FDA approved in the United States as of this writing. Drs. F. Frauscher and G. Bartsch, in their 2006 presentation at the 92nd Scientific Assembly of the Radiologic Society of North America noted that this simple technique improved vessel detection allowing for targeting these areas and finding more cancers. In 3446 patients screened with this modality, the overall cancer detection rate was 32%. However, 1/3 of tumors occurred in men with a PSA between 2.0-3.9 ng/ml and these were men in the lower age groups.

Ironically, a French exchange physician, Dr. Olivier Lucidarme, developed an ultrasound agent in 1999 at the University of California San Diego. Since it was not FDA approved, he returned to Paris, France and is perfecting this exciting modality, demonstrating the microcirculation in tiny cancers and detecting these before other imaging technologies. Dr. Kenen et al, in the IEEE *Trans Med Imaging*

Journal (2011), reported a way to quantify the diffusion of contrast by computers to assess the microvascularity of a tumor and correlate it with cancer angiogenesis. The same has successfully been done for vascular analysis of dangerous melanoma skin cancer.

A colleague of Dr. Lucidarme, Dr. Francois Cornelis, from Pellegrin Hospital in Bordeaux, France will be practicing in New York as a fellow at Memorial Sloan Kettering Cancer Center from 2013-2014. Dr. Cornelis wrote the CEUS chapter in my medical textbook *Image Guided Prostate Cancer Treatments* (Springer Berlin 2013) and has graciously consented to work with the Biofoundation For Angiogenesis Research and Development to extend the use of this technology to imaging metastatic glands. Another expert researcher, Dr. Ximena Wortsman, author of *Dermatologic Ultrasound With Clinical And Histologic Correlations* (Springer Berlin 2013), has advanced the technology of CEUS to the study of metastatic lymph nodes from the most deadly cancer, malignant melanoma. This truly lethal disease metastasizes widely and involves lymph nodes in all parts of the body. The current method of staging tumor spread of melanoma involves a biopsy of the lymph nodes that may be involved. This is not unlike the random prostate biopsy although it involves giving the patient an injection of radioactive tracer, then using a Geiger counter to follow the disease, and finally surgical removal of the node(s) under general anesthesia. A special use of CEUS to verify that a potentially involved "sentinel" node is unaffected by metastases is described by Dr. Wortsman on page 270 of her book. This may save many patients from unnecessary lymph node biopsies. Dr. Wortsman will join our multicenter group to be overseen by the Mount Sinai Medical Center in the study and development of this technique.

Another use of this technology is to predict treatment outcome. Dr. Y. Kono, in the 2007 *Journal of Vascular and Interventional Radiology*, found blood flow regression to occur as early as two days after successful intra-arterial chemotherapy. Such results are usually available after three months by CT and MRI exams. Results were based on liver cancers but portend well for evaluating therapeutic outcome for any vascular tumor. This minimally invasive modality may reduce the need for biopsy sampling to ensure a clinically effective endpoint. A 2007 article in *Journal of Urology* by Drs. Mitterberger et al (Medical University of Innsbruck, Austria) showed that contrast enhanced color Doppler biopsies showed higher grade tumors better than routine biopsies. While this contrast agent is not FDA cleared, it appears that the latest generation of power Doppler units which became available in the US in 2007 will prove an accurate substitute. From Holland,

Drs. Smeenge, Laguna and de la Rosette, in the new textbook *Imaging And Focal Therapy Of Early Prostate Cancer* (Thomas Polascik MD, ed., Springer 2013), note that very few articles exist on this subject and see the need to find a clinical niche for this modality. What has emerged is the verification of thermal treatment (heat/cold) results. For example, in the HIFU treatment of a tumor, CEUS absent flow signals indicates no viable tissue. Dr. Olivier Rouviere, one of the developers of the French HIFU technology, uses this to verify that lack of vessel existence starts as early as minutes after the treatment and has lasted up to 45 days in his 2011 study, published in the journal *Radiology*. Focal Laser Ablation (FLA) has similarly been studied with CEUS before, during and after the thermal treatment. A 2009 Canadian study showed that the destroyed area had no viable blood flow, and, as more laser treatment occurred, the newly treated regions lost their vascularity. These findings were confirmed by contrast MRI.

French radiologists, Drs. A. Cornelis and J-M. Correas, have shown that CEUS is positioned to become the primary modality for detecting prostate cancers of significance, since the test does not use ionizing radiation or potentially dangerous intravenous injections. The safety of this procedure has been verified over the past decade and the contrast agent is now FDA approved for cardiac studies.

Physicians are now using this off label[10] in the United States to diagnose tumors in all areas of the body. The quantification of micro-blood flow in disease may offer a better functional indicator of tumor aggression and metastatic potential. Dr. Richard Barr presented a variety of clinical uses for this technology at the 2012 American Institute of Ultrasound in Medicine in his ten years experience in the United States with off label media.

Sono-elastography

European and Japanese investigators have developed a novel way to show the toughness of tissue using special ultrasound properties showing the elasticity of investigated organs. Cancer tissue is usually firmer than benign tumorous tissue which is, in turn, harder than normal tissue. When I place a needle to biopsy a cancer, I can feel the gritty nature of the malignant area during the

---

10   Note: Merriam-Webster defines "off label" as referring to "an approved drug legally prescribed or a medical device legally used by a physician for a purpose (as the treatment of children or of a certain disease or condition) for which it has not been specifically approved (as by the United States Food and Drug Administration)." For example, Botox® was originally approved by the FDA for the treatment of facial spasms in 1989, and then in 2002 for diminished facial lines. Legal off label uses now include wider medical applications.

aspiration or biopsy process. A needle inside a benign lesion often has a rubbery, softer feel. Normal tissues tend to have little resistance to the needle passage. Palpation to assess a tumor has been part of medicine since Hippocrates. The measurable quality of firmness in diseased tissue was studied over 200 years ago by a British physician, Thomas Young, and is related to the deformation of an area when subjected to physical stress forces. Elastography essentially uses computers instead of fingers to examine abnormal areas using Dr. Young's basic principles.

Elastography, using sonographic equipment and special computer analysis, was perfected by the Laboratory of Waves and Sound in Paris and has been performed in breast cancer diagnosis for several years with significant success. Equipment developed by the Curie Institute in Paris is being used to measure the severity of liver cirrhosis (scarring) and healing in response to medical treatment. This has been so accurate that is has replaced liver biopsies to ensure improvement has occurred. Drs. L. Pallwein and F. Frauscher in their presentation at the 2006 Radiologic Society of North America, and paper in *Current Opinions in Urology* (2007), observed this was a useful but as yet not highly specific diagnostic test. However, European studies are showing that sonoelastography-guided biopsies target the cancer 2.8 times more accurately than without this technology. A 2007 article in *Journal de Radiologie* by Dr. Anne Tardivon from the Curie Institute showed a 96.7% negative predictive value in breast tumors, meaning that minimally suspicious tumors could be watched rather than biopsied. This technique may eventually be used to stage the spread of cancer. Drs. Pallwein and Frauscher, who use the same ultrasound unit I have, reported in the 2007 ECR meeting many false positives (275 out of 533 suspicious areas) yet feel it is truly valuable as more experienced is gained. However, the stiffness of the seminal vesicles by cancer infiltration and tumor penetration through the capsule had higher accuracy when compared with MRI findings. Many ultrasound equipment manufacturers are now developing a more sophisticated version specific for the prostate. A 2010 study in *Ultrasound in Medicine & Biology* showed that there are new variations of elastography (just like there are 6 different formats for Doppler ultrasound) and that the diagnostic accuracy in the prostate is increased 250% with this modality. As this non invasive method is being further improved, work is being done in MR Elastography[11]. The future of both technologies looks promising.

---

11   Li. S et al in 2011 Acta Radiol p.354-8

To take innovation to another level, researchers (engineers, radiologists, etc.) merged elastography with radiofrequency ablation (RFA). Heat-ablated tissues are stiffer (less elastic) than normal tissue. Drs. Lee and Varghese in the 2003 *American Journal of Radiology* report using sonoelastography in real time to confirm effectiveness of thermal treatments. Afterward, their images correlated very well with the pathologic specimen of the treated tissues. The real-time assessment with sonoelastography is essentially instantaneous and avoids lost time waiting to verify success by CT or MRI scans days or weeks later. Since the success of the procedure can be assessed at the time of treatment, additional ablation may be performed if necessary. Dr. Konig in 2005 *Journal of Urology* used elastography to guide prostate biopsies in a series of 404 patients and demonstrated an 84% success rate. This two-year study used the same 3D PDS unit that I have had for 4 years; however, no comparison was made between the success of the power Doppler function vs. the elastography feature.

Dr. David Cosgrove, radiologist from the Imperial College of Medicine, London, presented work at the 2012 JFR, Paris noting that breast imaging with this modality is 99% accurate in a large two year study. This means that English women may be spared unnecessary biopsies and agonizing waiting for the results with a simple non x ray exam. I am presenting prostate MRI and Doppler papers at the 2014 American Institute of Ultrasound in Medicine April 2014 and will update my readers in a newsletter about progress in the fusion of MRI, ultrasound and elastographic technologic breakthroughs.

HyperSpectral Imaging (HSI)

This non invasive technology was originally used to penetrate the earth's crust to find oil deposits or analyse contaminants in the atmospheric air we breathe by the application of long wavelength electromagnetic waves. Using short wavelengths, such as visible light, images of tumors of the skin, breast, prostate and lymph nodes have been obtained. In the same fashion that 3D-PDS was first used industrially, HSI now has medical patents for the detection of cancerous lymph nodes (glands) and malignant melanoma detection. The skin can be imaged with a special camera taking pictures in seconds for analysis. Internal organs, such as the prostate and esophagus require tailored probes to illuminate and record these tissues for analysis. Additionally, oxygen concentrations in blood may be measured and the change in oxygen levels becomes an indicator or treatment success. The non invasive and cost effective nature of HSI suggests more clinical use in the near future.

PhotoAcoustic Imaging (PA)

Similar to the previous technology that uses light to produce reflected images, PA uses high intensity light and/or lasers to transmit energy into the tissues which generates ultrasound waves that are detected by an ultrasound transducer. This is currently not FDA approved but has been extensively used in non-invasive animal testing since it images small organs and provides oxygen concentration data. This is being used in medical centers outside the USA with success. While the test is non-invasive, the precautions of using laser illumination and the high cost of the equipment mean that it is not ready for prime time clinical use this decade.

3 Tesla MRI (3T-MRI)

Until recently, most MRI scans were performed under a magnet using a magnetic field strength of 1.5 Tesla (1.5T MRI). In the past few years higher magnetic field strengths have become available, so 3.0 Tesla (3T MRI) systems are now being utilized. The higher field strength shortens the exam time so fewer minutes are spent inside the magnet tube—a blessing for the claustrophobic. While some increase in resolution is usually obtained, the systems are not yet fully optimized as of this writing for examining the prostate. Unfortunately, tiny pieces of metal in the eye or other parts of the body that would not be affected by a 1.5T magnet, may be pulled toward a higher field strength system, possibly resulting in injury to the patient and conceivably causing blindness. 7T units are currently being tested on animal prostates with impressive results.

Contrast enhanced MRI (DCE-MRI)

Contrast agents can be used to enhance targeted organs and disease conditions. Paramagnetic gadolinium contrast can be injected intravenously to highlight cancer detection during the MRI exam. This is called contrast enhanced (CE) or dynamic MRI sequencing. While this has improved tumor visibility, computer-aided detection has been more advantageous in determining tumor aggression. Developed by an Israeli scientist, Hadassa Degani PhD, we have been using the process in breast and prostate cancer patients for ten years. Contrast flows through the veins and diffuses into and out of the prostate, called the wash-in and wash-out principle. Abnormal wash-in/wash-out occurs in cancers due to the abnormal vessel caliber and increased vascularity that results in vascular permeability (leaky vessels) and detectable contrast in the tumor space. The computer program color-codes the cancer red and the normal tissue blue). Color coding is quantifiable and may be used as a baseline for treatment. This is especially important in patient care since the effect of chemotherapy may be demonstrated in some breast and prostate cancers within a few days following the first treatment.

Computer-aided full time point MRI (FTP-MRI)

Another MRI modality that also uses color coding is FTP-MRI (full time point MRI), previously mentioned in Chapter 4. We have been following up high grade prostate cancers within three to seven weeks of treatment with 3D PDS and FTP-MRI. We see dramatic reversal of hypervascularity in most cases within that time frame. If a therapeutic result is not achieved within 12 weeks in the prostate tumor, consideration is given to other medical management. Sequential 3D PDS and FTP-MRI are optimizing treatment decisions. Clinicians are beginning to favor this accurate color coded imaging modality over the S-MRI technologies since we are able to detect the small tumors sometimes missed by current spectroscopic protocols. In our practice, the addition of FTP MRI has permitted the avoidance of the ER (endorectal) coil, the use of which is both time consuming and uncomfortable. Colorized FTP MRI images are usually available within an hour or two of the scan sequence. In similar manner to the 3D PDS imaging, blood flow parameters of MRI are being studied and proving clinically effective. At our center, we are using the proven 3D Doppler technology to calibrate the newer computer aided MRI flow sequences. As the FTP MRI is improved, new secrets of blood flow within cancers may be revealed so that the 3D PDS imaging may also be improved.

Lymph node MRI (LNMRI)

Part of the reason for treatment failures with pelvic cancers is the presence of small nodes and hidden nodes that cannot be visually identified by the surgeon. Some or all of these may contain cancerous cells. Drs. Harisinghani and Saksena presented three papers at the 2007 American Roentgen Ray Society (ARRS) meeting demonstrating the new technique of MRI imaging lymph nodes distinguished between unremarkable glands and cancer filled nodes. Under MRI guidance, abnormal findings were biopsied. This resulted in the discovery of unsuspected cancer spread, thereby altering treatment protocol. Over three percent (3.7%) of patients in the study were shown to have small-to-medium (4-8mm) perirectal nodes (invisible nodes around rectum). Since these nodes are not evaluated during routine surgical removal of the lymph node chains, either MRI and/or 3D ultrasound imaging becomes the diagnostic modality of choice, provided it includes a special unit designed to evaluate the perirectal space. Newer contrast agents for this purpose are currently under investigation in Europe with great accuracy in early trials.

New MRI blood flow technologies

Given the high specificity of 3D PDS cancer detection when abnormal blood flows appear on images, MRI researchers have been improving blood flow techniques that point to tumors. The essence of MRI detection of cancer is "leaky vessels:" abnormal vessels leaking the injectable medium that marks the tumor tissues. The latest protocols have been highly successful in demonstrating the cancer and its extracapsular spread and were reported in the 2009 conference of the ARRS by Drs. Bard, Liebeskind and Melnick; and by myself at the 2007 American Society of Clinical Oncology. Advances in computer analysis of flow data are improving this reliable technology. Since there are false positives in inflammation, abnormal flow states are correlated with other MRI parameters in addition to 3D PDS.

Positron emission tomography (PET scans) also known as PET/CT

PET scan technology available in the US has had limited value in prostate applications, even though it is being widely used for other cancer detection. This is because PET utilizes a radioactive isotope that is injected into the vein and localizes in abnormal tissues. Since this is excreted by the kidneys, it fills the bladder and obscures the prostate. More importantly, many prostate cancers and their metastatic sites grow more slowly than most other more aggressive cancers and have a lower uptake of the isotope resulting in decreased sensitivity. Advances by Dr. Jean-Noel Talbot (Paris, France) and others have furthered the diagnostic use of this modality within the prostate. CT imaging can produce an overlay providing anatomic triangulation of the diseased organs; it uses a glucose (sugar) based isotope and is called FDG PET scan. Outside the U.S., a PET radioactive isotope using *choline* instead of glucose is called FCH PET or choline-PET scan. As the technology improves, further prostate applications will likely be developed.

Diffusion Weighted MRI (DWI) including Whole Body Studies

This technology is a rapid scan that shows restricted flow of water molecules which is due to a more aggressive tumor. It is an accurate assessment of malignancy by itself and may be used throughout the body to find metastases. Since this is a non radioactive test, it may be used instead of the radio-isotope PET/CT scan.

Prostate size reduction before definitive cancer treatment

As a rule of thumb, the smaller the prostate gland the better the effectiveness of localized cancer treatments. Before initiating HIFU treatment, European urologists who use this ablation technology first reduce the size of the gland by TURP (transurethral resection of the prostate). They have shown the smaller the gland the shorter the treatment. Also the chance of urinary obstruction is lessened because the postoperative gland produces less swelling around the urethra. This shortens the recovery time as well. Over 1000 cases have been successfully performed with this pretreatment size reduction. Radiation and hormone therapies are also used to shrink the prostate volume prior to certain treatments.

One unfortunate side effect presented at the 100th Annual AUA Meeting in 2005 was that the TURP procedure had a high association with painful ejaculations after men had this surgery. A new technique offers the benefits of a smaller prostate for definitive cancer treatments but with less trauma. In 2000, researchers from the Department of Surgery at the Catholic University Hospital in Rome began injecting *botulinum neurotoxin type a* (Botox®) into the prostate to improve symptoms of benign enlargement. During the course of a year, prostate volume decreased by half and symptoms improved. This was performed by manual injection without ultrasound guidance. Studies were performed by the Mayo Clinic, as well as the University of Perugia Medical Center (Italy) using ultrasound guided injections of Botox®. No significant side effects were reported, and the intervention appears to be harmless yet effective.

Drs. Guercini, Giannantoni and myself presented a paper verifying this conclusion, based on our own work, at the 2005 AUA Meeting, before 10,000 urologists. We specifically noted the sometimes remarkable reduction in prostate volume of this procedure. Indeed, one of our patients from England dramatically reduced his gland size from 130 to 40 cc (6x normal down to 2x normal) in just a month. This observation prompts the question: could injection of *botulinum neurotoxin* be a way to reduce the size of an enlarged prostate gland prior to HIFU, surgery or radiation? This could rapidly reduce the size of the prostate so that cancer treatments will be more rapidly available, and have a higher likelihood of success. It currently takes 3-6 months before hormone treatments reduce the size significantly, but these have unpleasant side effects—much like a man going through female menopause because the drugs deprive the body of testosterone production. In the case of a man with a high grade cancer and a 60 cc prostate, a *botulinum neurotoxin* injection that shortened the reduction time to a month would prove miraculous. The use of ultrasound guidance permits injections to avoid the site of the cancer and decrease the risk of cancer cells spreading outside the prostate while delivering a therapeutic dose to the site of the benign enlargement. The 3-D/4-D ultrasound probe allows the most accurate positioning of the needle. Since needle placement is optimized, we are able to use a small (22 gauge) needle that is virtually painless during the insertion and injection phases. This pretreatment shrinkage can only make minimalist treatments more effective. This procedure is still in clinical trials.

Antioxidant therapies are likewise proving effective in diminishing prostate size. One patient with a 900 cc prostate (think *grapefruit!*) shrunk the gland down to 300 cc within 8 months and has maintained the size between 250 to 340 cc for the last two years with this regimen. He claims the only trouble he has urinating is when he becomes constipated.

Radiofrequency ablation (RFA) and thermotherapies

Dr. Bruno Fornage, an Interventional Radiologist at the MD Anderson Cancer Center in Texas, has studied radiofrequency ablation (RFA) outside the usual guidelines. It involves running a high frequency electrical current through target tissues, and ablates (destroys) them by generating intense heat. While this technique has been successfully applied to tumors of the liver, kidney, lung, brain, and (in Europe) the prostate, Dr. Fornage studied small tumors of the breast and published his findings in the 2004 *Radiology*. Twenty-one patients with malignancies were treated with RFA prior to surgical mastectomy. The results of examining the specimens showed that this technique is both feasible and safe in tumors less than 2 cm in size. In Belgium, Drs. Zlotta, from the Erasme Hospital in Brussels and Dr. Michael Marberger, a Professor of Urology from Vienna, treated 15 prostate cancer patients using RFA. Their 1998 published results in the *British Journal of Radiology* show the destruction of the cancers was reproducible and controlled. While small tumors of the prostate may be treated with RFA with few side effects, it is a challenge to consider treatment of the entire gland due to the adjacent structures of the rectum, nerves and bladder. Perhaps the techniques developed for cryosurgery and HIFU to increase the space between the rectum and the prostate by saline injection may be applied to this evolving technology. If so, it would allow the more aggressive use of larger needles to treat the entire prostate and surroundings with acceptable complication rates.

Drs. Neeman and Wood, from the Diagnostic Radiology Department of the National Institutes of Health Clinical Center and the National Cancer Institute, published an article for *Techniques in Vascular and Interventional Radiology* (2002) discussing newer uses of RFA. Diagnosis and selection for RFA are critical. Small tumors that are isolated from major blood vessels, bowel, nerves and bladder make the best candidates.

RFA is a team procedure and consultation with surgical oncologists, pain control specialists and palliative care practitioners is useful in pre-procedure evaluation. For small and localized areas, local or intravenous anesthesia is useful, while for larger invasive regions, spinal or general anesthesia may be used. A post-op patient controlled analgesia (pain reliever) pump may be administered for large treatment sites. The 3-D sonographic imaging accurately allows placement of the metallic tines (that physically run the current through the tissue) in position, and the procedure may be completed in about 20 minutes for a 1 cm tumor. Vascular tumors successfully treated no longer show blood flows upon termination of the heating. A useful feature of this modality is that the entry path for the treatment needle may be cauterized upon exiting to destroy any malignant cells seeded in to the needle site. This access tract heating also controls bleeding. An anticipated complication in the prostate would be swelling that would prevent urination. This can be treated prophylactically with a Foley (penile) or suprapubic catheter. However, small tumors away from the urethra may not cause urinary obstruction, so the patient could be monitored for voiding difficulties in this situation. In May, 2005 an animal study by Dr. Nahum Goldberg (Dana Farber Cancer Institute; Harvard Medical School; Boston, MA) was published in *Radiology*. The article noted better tissue destruction if RFA was combined with intravenous chemotherapies. Currently RFA use in the prostate is FDA approved but still under investigation at many teaching centers.

Preparing to destroy a tumor's blood supply by imaging blood vessels

Angiogenesis or new blood vessel formation in tumors (from the Latin: angio = blood vessel, genesis = creation) plays a pivotal role in the development and progression of cancer. The high prevalence of cancer-induced growth of arteries and veins makes these vessels a logical target for cancer therapy. Antiangiogenesis therapy, that is, treatment to physically destroy the blood vessels supplying a tumor, has several theoretical advantages. First, the tumor blood vessels are generally more homogeneous than the tumor cells. Secondly, the lining cells of the vessels are stable so acquired drug resistance may be rare. Third, a partial damage to the lining cells may be enough to block blood supply to a tumor, resulting in growth inhibition or even shrinkage of the cancer. This treatment requires imaging the arteries and documenting changes in the blood vessels and its effect on the tumor. Without blood and oxygen supplied by these pipelines, a tumor cannot survive. The ability to demonstrate these vessels will not only improve diagnosis, but will further research and development of newer treatments.

The following are criteria for an ideal vascular imaging technique:

- Non-invasive
- Risk free
- Completed in less than 60 minutes
- No expensive monitoring required (no nursing or post procedure recovery expense)
- Free of ionizing radiation
- No danger to the kidneys—no dye (iodinated contrast) utilization
- Painless
- Applicable to all patients
- Objectively and easily performed
- Easy to interpret by trained personnel
- Cost effective
- Provide 3-D rendering of vascular anatomy

Arteriography, a radiographic technique using invasive catheters to inject dye by puncturing the artery, does not satisfy the above criteria except for accurate anatomic and physiologic information. The advantage of sonography is that it is quick, painless and void of radiation. The physician can see tiny blood vessels in the body. Angiogenesis evaluation by power Doppler has proven clinically significant in providing important prognostic information in patients with colon, gastric, ovarian and cervical cancers and in skin melanomas. Advantages (and disadvantages) are that it is both operator and equipment dependent. It requires a physician highly skilled in both ultrasound and urology for the prostate. The equipment varies widely in price and capability. Optimal equipment for the prostate has power Doppler and automated 3-D imaging features. Acceptable sonogram devices can image blood vessels as small as 0.6 mm in diameter and show the capsule of the prostate in three dimensions; devices that can image blood vessels between 1.5 and 0.6 mm are important because the vascular nature of aggressive prostate cancer is that they are generally supplied by arteries within this size range.

Excellent quality images with CT angiography and MR angiography are available in many medical centers. No puncture of the artery is necessary, though intravenous dye is required. Other modalities (contrast enhanced ultrasound, contrast enhanced CT, contrast enhanced MRI and diffusion MRI) have not yet been clinically helpful in this area. My colleagues and I are testing a new MRI vascular computerized imaging protocol, called FTP DCE-MRI, which is proving useful. Thus far, it appears that the optimal way to diagnose aggressive prostate cancer is by using 3-D Power Doppler Sonography (3D PDS). To go a step further, combining 3D PDS with DCE MRI allows almost immediate evaluation of the impact of thermal ablation on both the tumor and its blood supply, which may eliminate the need for post treatment multiple biopsies.

Antiangiogenic drugs

One way to stop blood circulation to a tumor is to prevent the vessels from developing. This is like tying a tourniquet around the artery. Angiogenesis is a process where a tumor sends out protein molecules to promote development of new blood vessels. These vessels then provide nourishment to the cancer, even as they allow malignant cells to spread throughout the body. The recently FDA approved colon cancer drug Avastin cuts off the supply line to the tumor. This antiangiogenesis effect was discovered accidentally after the horrible birth defects from the drug Thalidomide® which appeared to block blood vessel growth in the developing fetus. There are over 70 antiangiogenesis drugs currently in human cancer testing, and they rarely cause significant side effects in older individuals. According to William Li, President of the Angiogenesis Foundation in Cambridge, the notorious drug, Thalidomide (or its less toxic variants) may be the next product to receive FDA approval for stopping tumor growth. It has been intensively investigated as an anti-angiogenesis agent and proven effective in treating patients with multiple myeloma (common bone cancer in elderly patients) and Kaposi's sarcoma (aggressive skin malignancy common in AIDS patients).

A paper presented by Taiwanese radiologists, Dr. Chiun Hsu and associates, at the 2005 Radiologic Society of North America Meeting looked at the effect of Thalidomide on vascular liver tumors. Dr. Hsu had previously reported that low doses of Thalidomide induced tumor control in patients with highly aggressive liver cancer. Dr. Hsu chose to monitor Thalidomide treatments by using power Doppler sonography (PDS) without the 3D component. In his series of 44 patients treated with oral Thalidomide, 5 patients responded with clinically significant results. Of these responders, most had highly vascular tumors. The positive results of this study may be further enhanced in the liver and other organs by integrating local ablations such as RFA and HIFU. A downside to Thalidomide is the occurrence of deep venous thrombosis (blood clots in the veins that may go to the lungs) and peripheral neuropathy (nerve damage) that may be irreversible.

Studies are ongoing to decrease these side effects by adding other drugs in combination. The addition of Heparin (blood thinner) has improved patient tolerance as reported in the *Journal of Clinical Oncology* (July 2004). A study out of the National Cancer Institute, by Dr. A. Retter et al, suggested that this treatment would be optimally utilized in patients who have failed standard hormone treatments. Their paper presented at the 2005 Meeting of the American Society of Clinical Oncology showed the entire patient group in the trial sustained PSA declines by greater than 50%. Thalidomide is currently marketed under the brand name Thalomid. Newer varieties of this drug with fewer side effects are currently being developed. Combining drugs for a synergistic effect appears more potent than single agents used alone.

Physicians in the United States may, in the near future, treat prostate cancer through the newer emerging technologies of endo (inside) vascular (vessel) therapy. European centers are injecting chemotherapies directly into the cancerous tissues rather than administering this toxic treatment throughout the body by intravenous injection. The results by Dr. Ursula Jacob in Germany have been impressive in many patients. Her cancer control has been verified by follow up with 3D PDS and MRI protocols as well as reduction of the PSA and clinical findings.

Dr. Barry Stein at the International Symposium on Endovascular Therapy, 2004 gave a lecture entitled "New Concepts for a Modern Day Non-invasive Service" in which he claims that the report of a sonogram, CT or MR exam should contain a clinical assessment, including implications for possible endovascular management and treatment of the clinical problem. He feels that it is incumbent on the physician who images a cancer to offer the patient the benefit of the newer technologies over existing modalities. He says:

> *We would be remiss if we didn't and couldn't educate the general public and patients to safer and less expensive alternative technologies to investigate disease…Patients are naturally very receptive to embrace any pain free, cutting edge technology over old relatively morbid alternatives. It is extremely important to empower the patient with the knowledge of alternative diagnostic studies when faced with the need for an angiogram (arterial dye study).*

Said another way, the doctor who diagnoses the tumor could be the one to pursue treating it most effectively. It seems reasonable that the physician looking at a vascular prostate cancer would be the physician treating it. Logically, the tumor with high blood flow can be destroyed by antiangiogenesis drugs. Another method would be to simply cut off the blood supply. The artery supplying the tumor could be identified and blocked in some mechanical fashion and quickly assessed by 3D PDS and/or FTP MRI. Such blockage is called occlusion or embolization.

Arterial embolization (blocking blood flow) and related interventions

So, how can one plug a blood vessel? Everyone knows there are two ways to block a sink drain. Either shove something big inside the pipe, which will block flow immediately, or flush sticky food particles, like greasy rice and corn down the drain, which slowly obstruct it. Think of a hose running from a garden faucet as the artery that delivers blood to a cancer, and imagine it has smaller hoses branching off from it. A large object inside the artery will stop the flow at once. Smaller particles may not block the hose, but will clog its smaller branches. In medicine, this process is called "embolization."

Microspheres are small beads that were first used in 1960 to block abnormal blood vessels in the brain. They are often made from an acrylic co-polymer though other substances are also used. New microspheres of uniform size were developed in the mid 1990's to block dilated blood vessels and for preoperative embolization and devascularization of hypervascular tumors. The targeted embolization of benign uterine tumors (fibroids) is an FDA approved treatment. Tagging chemotherapeutics or radioactive materials to these spheres has produced good clinical results in liver cancers of the primary type and metastatic variety. Japanese physicians have used this technique for the last 20 years. The studies on uterine tumors showed that the dilated feeding blood vessels preferentially suck up the microspheres in what is called the "sump effect." German physicians are using these effectively in prostate cancer control.

A variation on this concept is being developed in Montreal at the Laboratoire de Nanorobotique (Nanorobotic Laboratory) using magnetized microparticles called nanospheres (nano = extremely tiny particles). Magnetic nanospheres may be directed using MRI fields to position a sort of "cluster time-bomb" inside the tumor. Radiofrequency waves of different types would activate them to produce local heat or release chemotherapeutics thereby destroying the cancer.

In 2004, the FDA approved microcatheters, tiny tubes that are easier to use to deliver the payload to a tumor. They deliver medications, microspheres or a stent balloon to the renegade blood supply with minimal damage to the arterial system through which it passes. This is also a possible delivery system for drugs such as Thalidomide with its anti-angiogenesis capabilities. A special variation of this is called the stiletto catheter. This is designed to penetrate the wall of a blood vessel and inject chemical products or thermal destructive energies into a tumor bed. The medical name is locoregional therapy, since it uses the artery as a conduit to the tumor and then performs ablative therapy on the cancer tissue outside the artery. This work has been successfully performed on liver tumors at The Johns Hopkins Hospital. Locoregional ablative therapy uses one or a combination of percutaneous ethanol injections (alcohol), radiofrequency ablation (heat), microwave energy (heat), laser beams (heat), high intensity focused ultrasound (HIFU) and acids such as acetic acid. Benign hypertrophy treatment of the prostate is now successfully performed with this modality.

Microwave hyperthermia

Microwave hyperthermia is a non-ionizing (not harmfully radioactive) form of radiation therapy that can substantially improve results from cancer treatment. In Phase III clinical trials where hyperthermia was combined with ionizing radiation treatments, hyperthermia improved 2-year local control of melanoma, complete response for recurrent breast cancer, 2-year survival for glioblastoma (aggressive brain cancer) and complete response for advanced cervical cancer, as compared to the use of ionizing radiation therapy alone.

Cancerous tumors are vulnerable growths of mutated cells that often require far more energy to survive than do normal cells. As cancer cells multiply unchecked, they can quickly outstrip the capacity of their existing blood vessels to supply enough oxygen and nutrients to support them. In response, malignant tumors stimulate growth of additional blood vessels. As shown in Chapter 3, these new blood vessels are mutated chaotic structures having odd sizes, loops and blind ends. Because of this irregular blood vessel structure and rapid tumor growth, there are often large areas where the tumor's blood supply is deficient.

Cancerous tumors that do not have an adequate blood supply become oxygen starved (hypoxic). They also become acidic because hypoxic tumors cannot adequately expel waste through the blood. These tumors can even experience wide fluctuations in blood flow as their unstable blood vessels periodically collapse, making them acutely oxygen deficient for periods of time. Oxygen starved cancer cells are difficult to kill with ionizing radiation (which creates oxygen radicals that attack tumor DNA) or chemotherapy (where blood transport is required to deliver the drug). Destroying blood/oxygen depleted cancer is a very high priority in cancer therapy because hypoxic cancer cells are especially dangerous, prone to metastasize and spread the cancer to other parts of the body.

Hyperthermia destroys cancer cells by raising the tumor temperature to a "high fever" range, similar to the way the body uses fever naturally when combating other forms of disease. Because the body's means of dissipating heat is through cooling from blood circulation, sluggish or irregular blood flow leaves cancerous tumors vulnerable to destruction at elevated temperatures that are safe for surrounding healthy tissues with normal, efficient blood cooling systems. Cancer cells are vulnerable to hyperthermia therapy particularly due to their high acidity caused by the inability to properly expel waste. Hyperthermia attacks acidic cells, disrupting the stability of cellular proteins and killing them. Hyperthermia is proving effective in increasing the effectiveness of radiation therapy, chemotherapy and surgery, since tumors tend to shrink after this treatment.

Gene therapy research is showing hyperthermia to be an activator to turn on new biological therapies, speeding gene production by thousands of times (heat mediated gene therapy). Hyperthermia plays an essential role in the development of anti-tumor vaccines that are based on heat shock. Research is showing hyperthermia to be an angiogenesis inhibitor, preventing cancer from inducing growth of new blood vessels to expand its blood supply.

Hyperthermia has further demonstrated use as a companion therapy for drug angiogenesis inhibitors, used in the final destruction of depleted cancer cells that survive blood starved conditions. Recent articles combining the use of *quercitin, resveratrol* and *ellagic acid* with localized hyperthermia are proving helpful in treatment of boney metastases. Hyperthermic states may be achieved simply by the use of therapeutic ultrasound units that treat muscle and pain disorders or more accurately by advanced radio or microwave generators. Dr. Paliwal, in the 2005 *British Journal of Cancer*, notes pretreatment of prostate cancer with ultrasound hyperthermia dramatically increases cell cancer death caused by the simultaneous administration of *quercitin*.

Hyperthermia has improved quality of life parameters for many patients. A recent study by the National Academy of Sciences has pointed out the shortcomings of the single-minded search for cancer cure while ignoring existing patients who need treatment for pain and other conditions associated with cancer. A substantial improvement in both palliation (pain relief) and durability of palliation has been observed when hyperthermia is added to ionizing radiation treatments. Some scientists have noted that hyperthermia stimulates the immune system, assisting patients in recovery from toxic cancer therapies such as chemotherapy and ionizing radiation. Even in situations where there is no hope for survival, hyperthermia may provide benefit through alleviation of such effects as bleeding, pain and infection. Hyperthermia is popular in Europe, but there has been a noticeable rate of tumor recurrence.

Irreversible electroporation (IRE)

Dr. Gary Onik, at the 2006 Annual Symposium of Interventional Therapy and the 2012 World Congress of Interventional Oncology, unveiled a novel ablation technique that uses nonthermal electromagnetic waves and may be competitive with current thermal ablation methodologies. The process is rapid and appears not to affect adjacent noncancerous structures such as nerves, bowel and bladder. The patented technology ablates a zone that can be imaged by 3D PDS as an echo-poor zone (dark) that turns echogenic (white) in 24 hours. This finding has not been confirmed by CT and MRI modalities. A surprising finding was that treated tumors produced an enhanced immunologic response to combat disease at the metastatic sites of the tumor. The human series so far is too small to admit this to the list of standard treatments, especially since a downside of the treatment is temporarily stopping the cardiac cycle in the human heart.

Dendritic cell immunotherapy

Immunotherapy uses the natural cellular immune system of the body to defend itself. The immune system consists of anatomic barriers such as the skin and acid in the stomach. If a foreign substance penetrates this shield, a second line defense is the inflammatory response. The last line of defense is the immune system which uses white blood cells to attack the invading organism. White blood cells include neutrophils which kill bacteria, eosinophils involving delayed response, monocytes (also called macrophages) which are scavengers, and lymphocytes which transfer cellular information and produce antibodies which inactivate or destroy foreign cells. When a tumor cell is noticed by the immune system, first a monocyte attaches and begins to digest the cell by breaking it into little pieces. The monocyte will then hand off the tumor remnants to other cells or transform itself into a specialized immune cell called a dendritic cell. This cell then migrates to a nearby lymph node which activates the army of lymphocytes (cytotoxic T lymphocytes) that attack the surface membrane of the cancer cells.

To be effective, the dendritic cell must be mature. Researchers are successfully developing juvenile dendritic cells into mature cells and "deploying" them into the body. There are studies showing its effectiveness in combating prostate cancer, lymphoma and malignant melanoma. At a 2006 think tank on evolving cancer therapies in New York, a highly successful treatment on prostate cancer patients was reported performed in the Philippines. The treatment seems to have few side effects and will be carefully monitored by the medical community. It is not FDA approved and is currently being performed outside the US in several centers with good results.

Nanoparticle therapies: thermal ablation and nanochemotherapy

Another spin-off of a military technology is being applied to cancer treatment. A battlefield repair system for body armor and other composite materials uses a resin saturated with nanoparticles (as many as 10,000 can fit on the end of a pin) that become heated when exposed to a magnetic field. The heated resin was molded and used to patch the broken materials before it cooled. The 2007 *Journal of Nuclear Medicine* cited an article by Dr. Gerald DeNardo and a worldwide group of authors participating in a University of California/Davis Medical School study of treating tumors in animals using this technique of heating nanoparticles labeled with antibodies specific to breast cancer cells. In the lab studies, it was found breast cancer cells were specifically killed when the culture dishes were exposed to antibody labeled iron oxide particles and an alternating magnetic field. After injecting trillions of nanoparticles of antibody-iron oxide and waiting three days for accumulation in the targeted cancer, magnetic fields instantly generated heat sufficient to kill the tumor without damaging nearby structures. Particles outside the tumor field were not significantly heated during the 20-minute treatment. No treatment side effects or toxicity was noted. It was felt that the treatment could be used to safely treat tumors anywhere in the body, as long as the circulating antibody-nanoparticle entity could get there. Since there is blood flow to all tumors, organ location would not matter. Human engineered antibodies exist for breast, prostate, lung, colon and ovarian cancers.

Another way to utilize nanoparticles is to integrate them with chemotherapy. An interesting property of microbubbles (water coated tiny air pockets) is that they can be made to rupture under a burst of ultrasound energy. This means that microbubbles may be steered into a tumor and then exploded by targeted sonography. Researchers at the University Hospital of Utah have been coating these objects with nanoparticles containing chemotherapeutic agents and permeating cancers with focal treatments. This work is encouraging and other similar pinpoint nanoparticle therapies are currently being developed with MRI technologies. A 2010 report in *European Urology* by Dr. Eggener shows that this work is promising and under intense study. A 2013 chapter in *Imaging And Focal Therapy Of Early Prostate Cancer* describes industry wide research for this concept in targeting nanomedicines for prostate cancer diagnosis and therapy.

Chemosensitivity testing and chemoembolization

Low dose targeted chemotherapy is possible if the right drug can be put in the right place. Dr. Thomas Rao in Switzerland has been using a blood assay to show the metabolic pathway of the cancer on a molecular-genetic basis. If a particular pathway is active, then it is more likely that a chemotherapeutic agent based on this pathway will be effective. The test analyzes and identifies circulating tumor cells in the blood stream. The test is only effective if circulating tumor cells are present. Also studied are the activity of the natural killer (NK) cells and modalities to increase their effectiveness. Based on these results, localized or whole body hyperthermia may be induced at the time the chemoembolic agents are injected into the artery feeding the tumor. High concentrations may be focally delivered sparing the normal tissues, thus generating better clinical outcomes and fewer side effects.

Gene therapy / molecular biology

Not so long ago, the future of genetic "bullets" looked rosy. However, a four year study from the US Human Genome Research Institute (involving 80 organizations around the world) is reshaping our mile posts. The long held view was each single gene in living organisms (humans, animals, plants, and bacteria) carried the information essential to construct a single protein specific to that molecule. Proteins are the building blocks and power systems that regulate cells, and by extension, living organisms. In the 60's, scientists discovered that a gene that produced one type of protein in one organism would produce a very close molecular clone in another entity. The standard medical application of this feature enabled insulin from pigs to be used safely by humans in the treatment of diabetes. It was assumed for years that a gene from a donor of any organism would predictably produce specified functions in another host organism. It was hoped genetic therapies would have a uniform effect with clear boundaries and discrete properties. Researchers depended on the fact that each sequence of DNA was linked to a single medical application, such as a predisposition to cancer, heart disease or diabetes.

The conclusion of this study by 35 international research groups showed a complex network of interactions between genes that is casting doubt on the "one gene, one protein" postulation. The assumption that genes operated independently must be rethought because overlapping functions of genetic material were shown to occur as the norm rather than as the exception. Genes are only one component of how a genome functions, with the other components not clearly understood. It seems that diseases are caused not by the action of a single gene, but rather by the interaction of multiple genes. For instance, a virulent form of malaria appears to involve interactions of 500 genes. Hopefully, another conclave of scientists will provide a clinical application manual for the newly discovered genetic variants in human treatment.

On a related note, the January 2005 issue of *Radiology Today* quotes Dr. Charles Cantor on genetic treatment of breast and prostate cancer. Dr. Cantor cites the December 2004 issue of *Cancer Research* that shows individuals with a certain bad gene have a 40% higher chance of developing breast and prostate cancer than those without this genetic defect. While the original study was designed to track breast cancer, it was found that it held true for prostate tumors. Since the bad genes are on the cell surface, Dr. Cantor predicts that new therapeutic opportunities will arise for breast and prostate cancer patients as drugs are made to target these sites. To date, there is no conclusive genetic treatment for prostate tumors.

Photodynamic therapy (PDT)

The use of light in cancer treatment, developed in the late 19th century in Germany, underwent a revival when the Japanese treated lung cancers in the 1980's. In 1998, the FDA approved this modality for microinvasive lung tumors. The patient is given an intravenous injection of a photosensitizer, which selectively accumulates in cancerous tissues. A laser directed at the tumor produces a free radical oxygen molecule that internally destroys tumor cells.

PDT has many names since it uses drugs along with light: photochemotherapy, photoradiation therapy, phototherapy and other variations of the name. Depending on the part of the body to be treated, the photosensitizing agent is either injected into the bloodstream or put on the skin. Over time, the drug is absorbed by the cancer cells. Light is then applied to the area to be treated causing the drug to react with oxygen forming a chemical that kills malignant cells. It also appears to destroy the blood vessels that feed the cancer, and alerts the immune system to attack the tumor. It is considered a less invasive procedure than surgery and can be repeated without systemic toxicity. Drugs for PDT have been approved by the FDA. The most common is porfirmer sodium (Photofrin) used against cancer of the esophagus and other sites that can be reached by light: lung, skin, vaginal and cervical cancers. The activating laser uses a low power light so it does not burn. Reports of successful light treatments of sensitized prostate cancer tissue have appeared sporadically. Dr. Nathan effectively treated local recurrence in a small study (2002 *Journal of Urology*) of radiotherapy failures; unfortunately, 4 of the 14 patients developed incontinence. Another side effect is the uptake of the photosensitizer in all the tissues, rendering patients acutely light sensitive for 6 weeks to 3 months. Finally, fiber optic cables must be inserted into the body to apply light to the tumor, necessitating sedation or general anesthesia.

A study by Drs. Pendse and Allen of the University College London presented at the 2007 AUA meeting studied a new light-activated drug (Tookad) developed at Israel's Weitzman Institute of Science. Tookad (the name in Hebrew means "the warmth of light") was injected into 27 patients whose biopsy-proven tumors were delineated by MRI. Under general anesthesia, light was diffused into the prostate. DCE-MRI taken one week post-therapy showed absent flow in the treatment sites which were followed up to 6 months using CE-MRI.

In the prostate, Tookad is harmless until exposed to light, usually by optical fibers. During PDT it appears to selectively constrict the blood vessels supplying the cancer, while leaving the healthy tumor intact. Drs. Avigdor Scherz and Yoram

Saloman have found the malignancy degenerates internally after the blood supply is cut off. Tookad is based on chlorophyll and has a shorter life span than other agents. Long term studies will show the overall effectiveness of this modality, but short term studies are showing encouraging results. Future advances may lead to the treatment of internal tumors such as esophageal and pancreatic cancer. Currently, there is limited use in the US with this modality in clinical settings.

MRI guided HIFU

High-intensity focused ultrasound (HIFU) was first suggested as a thermal ablative technique for brain tumors by Lars Leksell in 1949. He was frustrated by the ultrasound technology available at the time and went on instead to develop the gamma knife. In the 1950s, HIFU was developed to thermally ablate soft-tissue tumors. Thus, the technology has been around for more than 50 years. Though gaining popularity, it remains experimental and is currently not FDA-approved in the US. However, there are now published studies out of Europe and Japan reporting 10-year data, and interested readers can find these online.

With regard to MRI-guided focused ultrasound (MRgFUS), the most prevalent applications are the worldwide treatment of uterine fibroid tumors (benign growths) and bone metastases outside of the US. Now, a new device being used in Israel, the ExAblate® system, is being clinically tested for treatment of prostate cancer. It uses real time magnetic resonance imaging to visualize the tumor and surrounding structures, and to plan the energy delivery path of the focused ultrasound. A 2010 internet press release[12] reports on the "high intensity focused ultrasound beam which is delivered with millimeter precision to destroy the cancerous tumor without damaging surrounding tissue, which is the cause of most complications." The use of real-time 3D MR thermometry provides accurate closed-loop monitoring of the treatment outcome and ability to adjust the treatment according to specific patient physiology, in real time.

Galvanotherapy (GT)

Named in honor of the Italian pioneer in electricity, Luigi Galvani, this low voltage DC current therapy is a form of minimally invasive treatment used primarily in Germany and Scandinavia.

The voltage used is similar to a 9 volt battery and destroys malignancies by a combination of physical change and acceleration of immunologic activity at the

---

12   http://www.insightec.com/Prostate-Trials.html

tumor site. Combinations of this therapy with thermal therapies are available in Europe. One particular study out of Frankfurt, Germany, was published in 2007 in *Radiology*. It examined the results of treating 44 men with biopsy-proven prostate cancer using galvanotherapy, and was found to be a safe, well-tolerated treatment with reasonable cancer control. This is a minimally invasive technique, and more research is needed.

Laser assisted immunotherapy

Another possible new treatment should be considered since over 570,000 Americans will die of cancer this year. The technology is similar to Focal Laser Ablation described in CHAPTER 6 but adds the additional perspective of boosting the immune system to target metastatic disease, according to the 2011 article by Drs. St. Denis and Aziz et al in *Photochemical and Photobiological Sciences*, Vol 10 pp 792-801. Cells are destroyed using a near-infrared laser beam that is aided by a photosensitizer (indocynanin green is FDA approved). To attack the distant tumor spread, after the initial cancer is lasered, an immune booster or "adjuvant" that activates the patient's natural cancer killing cells is employed. These adjuvants are not FDA approved and are being developed outside the U.S. Following treatment of the primary tumor, the adjuvant is injected around the dying cancer. Further study is needed of this non surgical approach that may eventually be used to create vaccines to find and disable metastatic disease.

Future research

The nature of honest medical investigation is that surprises (pleasant and unpleasant) often occur. Innovation is risky. The art of medical innovation is to generate new uses for the unexpected. Simply put, "When life hands you a lemon, take sugar and ice and make lemonade." Hopefully researchers will have the integrity to identify early side effects as well as related possibilities of their discoveries. Proponents of a discovery may succumb to tunnel vision regarding the benefits of their product. Many drugs approved by the FDA and hyped on television commercials have been pulled off the market as life threatening problems became too apparent to dismiss.

Some unintended (and potentially dangerous) consequences of new developments may occur, even as long as a half century later. For example, the drug penicillin that saved my life as a child suffering with pneumonia eventually led to the creation of "superbugs" that are virtually unkillable. How did this happen? Antibiotics were truly miracle drugs that destroyed microbes. Not well understood for years was the genetic material responsible for conferring antibiotic resistance passed easily between different types of bacteria. The overprescribing of antibiotics for every ailment, especially the common cold, which is viral in nature, has created germs that are resistant to a class of antibiotic treatments. This has led to development of ever more powerful types of antibiotics which results in more strains of stronger bacteria. We are at a point where some bacteria are more powerful than the existing pharmaceutical products. While no one envisioned this scenario, hindsight shows the need to anticipate and monitor aftereffects.

Unexpected positive side effects may occur, too. Men taking antioxidant preparations notice healthier skin in addition to improved tumor response. Another surprising consequence was their medicine began quickly disappearing. It turned out that the wives started using their husbands' herbal formulations for erectile function support to attain smoother skin for themselves. Apparently, a widely-used drug that makes some thing hard can soften the skin in patients with advanced psoriasis. Dr. Mark Lebwohl, chairman of the Dermatology Department at Mount Sinai Medical Center in New York, has found the compounds in Viagra to be helpful in various skin pathologies.

Clearly, an open mind to any and all therapies, combined with well designed clinical trials, will further advance cancer survival and improve quality of life. Patients, the end users of modern technology, can be helpful in documenting and reporting unusual happenings. The team of patient, physician and scientist together can build a healthier future for mankind. Proven technologies may be further developed while problematic modalities may be earmarked for overhaul or discarded before they produce more harm. Also, many medical discoveries are published daily in prestigious scientific journals or presented at major specialty conferences without these findings being made available to the general public. The sheer volume of new findings has inundated physicians and confused patients. Our challenge is to ferret out important ideas and bring these to the attention of the medical community and patients likely to benefit from the treatment. Medical history demonstrates that administrative committees do not make discoveries. Rather, breakthroughs occur when individuals committed to change think outside the box and work outside the prevailing dogmatic principles. To paraphrase a quote: We will not have the land of the free if we are not the home of the brave. In other words, we must take risks and innovate if we are to fully harvest the fruits of scientific research.

CHAPTER 10

BOOSTING THE BODY'S DEFENSES

Let food be your medicine and your medicine be your food.
—Aristotle

Aristotle's quote reminds us that healing wisdom is sometimes simplicity itself. This chapter is basically a pep talk on long-established ways to maximize your good health, improve poor health, and even heal disease. A starting point in conquering cancer may be to realize that there is a myth to curing cancer. Perhaps certain cancers are a natural part of aging and must be dealt with accordingly in a demystified reality. Perhaps some are the result of an imbalance in the body. The combination of alternative healing with 21ˢᵗ century progressive medicine offers new hope and realistic choices for cancer victims. The data throughout the book shows clearly that we have not won the fight against prostate cancer. Cancer research funding is at extraordinarily generous levels, but still we cannot buy a cure for cancer. Until we identify the elusive cause(s) of cancer, develop ways to prevent them, and establish therapeutic methods that are not only effective but also kind to patients, learning to live harmoniously with cancer and other disabling illness is a creative response. Alternative healing provides such an opportunity.

Alternative medicine is coming of age with traditional practitioners who are witnessing the repeated successes of complementary medicine on cancer patients. As with other patient-driven trends, a powerful current is building, and it's always easiest to navigate a river by going with its flow. When I read the MRI report on a knee in an older patient (degenerative arthritis, torn meniscus, suprapatellar effusion, ACL edema, posterior cruciate tear, tibial cartilage loss, osteophyte formation, cartilage degeneration and internal bone cysts—all in one area) I am surprised that the patient standing in front of me could even walk, much less still play tennis during which activity he had just injured himself. I then ask the patient where he hurts, he points to one spot. I show him with the sonogram a partial tear in a ligament that can be healed with physical therapy and rehabilitation. But the multiplicity of problems in his knee is the result of years of under-informed choices and habits. In addition to physical therapy, this individual could benefit from lifestyle changes in keeping with complementary medicine. Adding better nutrition, natural supplements, acupuncture, stress management, reasonable exercise for his age, and meditation can improve not just his knee, but his entire physical, mental and emotional being for optimum wellness as he ages—and perhaps add years of good quality life, much as my father experienced after he managed his cardiovascular health through diet. A multidisciplinary approach that integrates all healing modalities for a particular patient is both good medicine and good business, as today's complementary trends will certainly influence future clinical practice.

For the last twenty years, I have been following patients with proven cancers who have been successfully treated for their disease. Some were told by senior physicians at major medical center to get their affairs in order, only to come to me for follow up scans that shock them. They are stunned not by the hopelessness of their situation, but rather by the significant regression of their disease thanks to complementary therapies. I advise my patients to try a treatment that they consider optimal for their lifestyle. We schedule a follow up visit to see if the therapy is effective by using the new scan as an interval comparison with the last 3D PDS study. An example is JW, a college professor, age 43, who came to me a year ago with a "feeling something was wrong in his pelvis." I scanned the prostate with sonogram and found a highly vascular, aggressive region at the base. The MRI confirmed the same findings of a tumor next to, but not involving the seminal vesicle. He wanted to try complementary medicine, but because of his relative youth and the seriousness of the tumor, I advised him to be biopsied at his university hospital. A week and 10 biopsies later, no cancer was found. He went on a complementary treatment as if he had cancer and the blood vessels disappeared 14 days later on a rescan. Six month follow up showed no tumor and he stopped his treatment unilaterally of his own volition without telling anyone. A one year follow up sonogram showed return of the original cancer with spread to both sides and extension out of the prostate. He refuses to have another biopsy and no is no longer a candidate for focal therapy. He is taking out a loan for whole gland HIFU because he is unwilling to risk losing his potency as he has recently remarried.

Naturopathic healers feel cancer is an outgrowth of a poisoned body and a depleted immune system. A 2005 book by Mitchell Gaynor, MD entitled *Nurture Nature Nurture Health* discusses the environmental impact on health. He cites a class of compounds called "xenoestrogens" which are estrogen mimicking chemicals found in plastics, wood preservers, cleaning solvents, pesticides, herbicides, PCBs used in electric insulators or dioxins and furans that result from burning municipal and toxic wastes. Apparently, more than 3200 chemicals are added to food and the EPA showed that 7.1 billion pounds of 650 industrial chemicals are found in our water and air. Linking contamination of our food chain with cancer, Dr. Gaynor feels that these estrogen mimicking compounds, which are associated with the onset of breast cancers, are contributing factors in men's prostate cancers. Synthetic hormones (estradiol and progesterone) implanted in cattle to increase their weight produce estradiol levels twenty times higher than normal in some meat products. A similar chemical, bisphenol, appears in many common plastic products-from food wrap to water bottles, and leaches out into liquids we drink. Bisphenol has another dangerous feature: the body registers it as a chemical hormone similar to those used in clinical hormone therapies, therefore rendering standard hormonal treatments less effective. Lastly, the zinc necessary for optimal prostate health is neutralized by metal pollution of lead and cadmium released from burning power plants and hazardous waste incinerators. What are we doing to our bodies—and more to the point, what can we do about it?

Food as preventative medicine

Nutritious foods are perhaps the easiest and most natural way to protect the body. Nutrient dense fruits and vegetables are more bioavailable than nutrients packaged in pills. This means that the body utilizes the vitamins and minerals and antioxidants more efficiently so they will be more effective in the healing process.

Cancer, which behaves opportunistically, may be a result of a body debilitated from stress and toxins. Clinical cancer may be a signal from the body that it is out of natural alignment, but good nutrition will go far in restoring internal balance and allowing the body to protect and heal itself. Good nutrition means choosing foods that are naturally rich in valuable nutrients and free from toxic chemicals. Certified organic foods are free of pesticide residues. Simple and seasonal locally grown products are often helpful. All produce must be washed with a diluted mixture of vinegar or bleach. Vegetables are the core of successful nutrition because they provide phytonutrients, antioxidants, soluble and insoluble fiber as well as essential minerals and vitamins. Books have been written on the beneficial effects of garlic which may be taken in the form of extracts. In tomatoes, the strong antioxidant lycopene deserves special attention for managing prostate disorders. A 2002 study by Dr. Giovannucci in *Experimental Biology and Medicine* showed that lycopene from tomatoes had a health benefit for prostate cancers, especially the more lethal forms. Work by Dr. Nicholas Gonzalez and Dr. Majid Ali has benefitted many cancer patients with nutraceutical formulations.

Nutrition is not just food; what's more important is how your body processes the food you eat. It also means eating and drinking foods in such a way that the tissues receive valuable nutrients and not unhealthy byproducts of inadequately digested foods and unhealthy intestinal bacteria. Whole grains are recommended, but not to excess. Wheat in particular contain glutens that are a major source of food sensitivity. A book by Dr. John E. Postley, *The Allergy Discovery Diet,* details the devastating effects of food sensitivities leading to allergic reactions which in turn compromise the body's immune system. Most grains and beans contain phytates and enzyme inhibitors that inhibit mineral absorption and weaken the intestinal enzymes, often producing flatulence.

Equally important is the maintenance of the body acid base balance. Vegetables (and most fruits) prevent the tissues from becoming overly acidic. High cellular acidity prompts the body to use up potassium, calcium and magnesium to buffer or neutralize the acid and realign with the normal slightly alkaline state. High acidity depletes the body of minerals and negatively impacts the immune system.

Hyperacidity has been associated with chronic infection, allergies and digestive difficulties. Avoiding sugar, processed cheese, meat and fried foods will help restore the natural alkaline state of the tissues. Fat is important in the diet since the cell membranes are made from fatty acids. A balance of omega 3/6/9 fatty acids may be obtained by skillful mixing of healthy fats and oils. Specifically, omega 3 and omega 6 compounds regulate inflammation in the body through their transformation into prostaglandins.

The process of digestion is another matter for consideration since food, drink and medicines have different properties affected by the acid environment and mix of good and bad microorganisms in the stomach and intestine. For example, protein breakdown takes much longer than for starch and vegetables. Older patients generate less hydrochloric acid which is essential for protein transformation into amino acids. Men with GERD (acid reflux or gastro-esophageal reflux) have reduced stomach acid due to treatment. Poorly digested food promotes the overgrowth of pathologic "bad" bacteria in the small intestine. The acidic and caustic byproducts of indigestion are called "endotoxins" and diffuse out of the intestine into the blood stream and thence throughout the body. Sugar and starch (which converts quickly back to sugar in the gut) feed the undesirable bacteria, producing even more internal toxins. Immune system tissues in the bowel and liver may be overloaded, reducing the overall immune response mechanism.

Supplements as preventative medicine

Therapeutic optimization would include supplemental vitamins, minerals, enzymes and antioxidants for an immune compromised patient. Melatonin, AHCC (active hexose correlated compound), Co-enzyme Q10, olive oil, omega-3 fatty acids have dietary anti oxidant value. Quercitin, resveratrol, ellagic acid, Ip6 (inositol hexaphosphate), TMG (trimethylglycine), selenium, zinc, plant sterols and pomegranate juice are proving valuable as a prostate health supplement. Green tea seems to be the most effective of the tea products. A clinical trial by Dr. Raymond Oyen, a professor at the medical school in Belgium, was presented in the 2008 Journal of Radiology. He observed that a plant sterol and antioxidant diet, including vitamin E, soy products and selenium, controlled many patients with precancers (PIN) and true cancers. Recent reports of Co-enzyme Q 10 are showing effectiveness in stabilizing prostate and breast cancers. Cancer researchers, Drs. Howenstine and Judy, are anecdotally documenting significant tumor regression. Dr. William Judy studied 30 patients with prostate cancer no longer inhibited by hormones and placed them on 500 mg of Co-enzyme Q 10 daily with substantial reduction in PSA levels.

Antioxidants as preventative medicine

What do antioxidants do? That depends on many factors, so let's review the terms:

- Antioxidants – molecules that absorb or neutralize free radicals in our cells
- Carotenoids – yellow, orange and red pigments synthesized by plants and can be converted by the body into vitamin A
- Enzymes – proteins found in cells that catalyze biochemical reactions; the most common that fight oxidation are CoQ-10 and superoxide dismutase
- Flavonoids – free radical scavenging antioxidants found in many plants
- Free radicals – atoms or molecules possessing unpaired electrons that cause cellular damage
- Phytonutrients – chemicals in plants, including antioxidants
- Polyphenols – antioxidant pigments found in many plants.

Antioxidants neutralize free radicals, the oxygen based-based molecules that are a rogue by-product of normal body metabolism. Most commonly found in DNA, cell walls and interiors, free radical molecules differ from normal molecules in one significant respect: they contain an odd or unbalanced number of electrons. Normal, stable molecules have an even number of paired electrons, whereas, in free radicals, one electron is missing its partner. This imbalance makes the molecule highly unstable so it searches for another single electron and steals it from another normal molecule. The theft of an electron turns this molecule into a free radical which sets up a cascade of electronic theft producing oxidative damage or oxidative stress. This produces oxidative damage to the DNA causing mutations. In the same way, free radicals also damage the cell walls reducing their protective functionality. In other words, they hasten the "rusting" (or oxidizing) of the body, resulting in disease and premature aging.

There are two ways antioxidants disrupt this process:

1. Some substances break the chain reaction, decreasing the production of free radicals
2. Others donate electrons to the scavenging molecules, returning them to a stable state

The following dramatically increase the body's free radical level:

- Sun exposure
- Smoking
- Excess alcohol consumption
- Excess caffeine consumption
- Chronic stress
- Overeating—the more food metabolized, the more free radicals formed
- Undereating—quick weight loss diets burn fat more quickly, releasing free radicals

Our body has its own antioxidant cleanup system rendering free radicals harmless, but in today's world we may be straining it to its limits. We are exposed to toxins, eat processed foods (often on the run), lead stressful lifestyles, etc. All of these factors burden our bodies with a barrage of free radicals, so supplementing a healthy food plan with additional antioxidants is wise. While there exist thousands of known antioxidants, experts believe that hundreds of thousands may be eventually discovered.

Antioxidants come in animal, mineral and botanical sources. Animal cells manufacture the important enzymes Co Q-10, glutathione and super-oxide dismutase. These act by fighting free radicals and catalyzing chemical reactions that stabilize the free radicals. (Note: Our body also makes these substances, but acute imbalance or disease states require greater amounts for combating disease-causing agents.) Mineral sources include zinc, copper and selenium. These must be carefully balanced since overdosage of any one mineral may be harmful. Botanical sources are the vast majority of chemical defenses against free radicals. Vitamins A, C and E are especially useful. Vitamin A works by quenching free radicals. Vitamin C offers up free electrons to the molecules that crave them. Vitamin E prevents oxidation by breaking the free radical chain reaction.

Thousands more botanical antioxidants are called phytonutrients and fall into three categories;

a) Flavonoids, a group that currently includes more than 4,000 chemicals, are all purpose scavengers because they find free radicals and then neutralize them by donating electrons. Quercitin, found in vegetables, dark chocolate and fruit skins, is especially active in this function. A large subcategory is polyphenols and phenolic compounds found in grapes, blueberries, pomegranates, cherries, raspberries, cranberries, grains and black and green tea. Resveratrol occurs in minute quantities in red wine.

b) Lignans: from seeds, like flax and sunflower.

c) Carotenoids: found in tomatoes, carrots, watermelon and spinach. The two main antioxidants are lycopene and lutein.

A prostate-specific reason to use antioxidant supplements comes from the 2007 American Society of Clinical Oncology presentation of pathologist Dr. De Marzo (Johns Hopkins) and Dr. Nakai (Osaka University, Japan) entitled *Inflammation and Prostate Carcinogenesis*. PIN or *prostatic intraepithelial neoplasia* seems to be a precursor for invasive prostate cancer and is detected only by biopsy. The standard medical treatment for this condition is to watch and wait. Antioxidant treatments block inflammatory LOX (lipoxygenase) enzymes and may help prevent PIN from progressing to aggressive cancer. The relationship between antioxidant pathways and highly aggressive "interval cancers" is undergoing intensive study at this time. The use of combinations of Co-enzyme Q-10 and resveratrol containing antioxidants to control cancer and inflammation is published in *Dermatologic Ultrasound* (Springer New York 2013).

A caution about soy and saw palmetto

Soy has been championed as a healthy alternative to animal protein. It is true that the Japanese eat soy and have lower rates of breast and prostate cancer but they have a higher incidence of stomach cancer. In addition to difficulty in digestion, soy contains protease inhibitors that reduce the efficiency of the digestive pancreatic enzyme trypsin. Dr. Nicholas Gonzalez, a New York City cancer specialist, cautions his patients about eating soy products since he feels pancreatic digestive enzymes are an important anti-cancer entity. Soy beans are high in phytic acid, contained in the hulls of the seed, and block absorption of essential minerals, such as calcium, copper, iron, magnesium and zinc in the intestinal tract. Clearly, soy isoflavones exert hormone effects in the human body, but the overall safety in cancer patients has not been established.

A study of *saw palmetto* by the University of California by Dr. Avins and presented at the 2006 AUA meeting underscored the fact that the extract did not improve flow or urinary symptoms on the standard 160 mg dose twice a day. More troublesome is the understanding that most of this plant material comes from central Florida in a section that has been designated a toxic waste site. This contamination may explain the increased incidence of hepatitis in patients who take this plant sterol.

The need to bolster the immune system

Malignant cell mutations occur within the body tissues continually and are regularly extinguished or inactivated by the body's defense mechanisms. Cancer cells are held in check by the immune system, which is the body's natural defense system. The immune system is made up of organs (like the skin and stomach) and cells (like white blood cells) that protect the body from dangerous agents. Lymphocytes (white blood cells) that kill cancers are called B cells, NK (natural killer) cells and T cells. These defensive cells attach themselves and kill anything foreign to the body. Other cells remove the inactivated cancer cells and the liver, kidney, lungs and digestive system ultimately discharge them from the body. Complementary medicine seeks to boost the immune system, and treat the underlying cause that disabled the body's natural defenses and allowed a tumor to grow. Immune system dysfunction sets the stage for cancer growth, and stress is a key culprit that saps this vital force, keeping it from successfully attacking and disabling newly formed tumor cells.

Stressors and stress

"I'm under so much stress!" bemoans the good man or woman who commutes two hours per day, works more 40 hours per week at a high pressure job, has a social life and family, donates volunteer time, etc. It would be more accurate to say, "I have so many stressors!!!" Stressors and stress are not the same. **Stressors** are the external events (or the internal thoughts and feelings about them) that jumpstart a chain reaction in our bodies. **Stress** is what happens next to our bodies. Suddenly, our normally balanced physical relationship of breath rate, heart rate, muscle relaxation, calm digestion, and so on goes into overdrive thanks to an onrush of neurological and biochemical mechanisms. These mechanisms are survival mechanisms as ancient as life itself, and originate in the earliest core of our brain: the limbic system. We have them in common with all creatures that have a central nervous system. When faced with threat, they are designed to impel fight, flight or temporary immobilization. Those preconscious survival strategies are hardwired within us: think of a prehistoric man being suddenly confronted by a dangerous predator—how much adrenaline will it take to generate an immediate reaction without losing precious seconds to think about it? Today's "predators" are rarely physical threats, but the circumstances of our rushed lives result in states of low-grade anxiety, even bordering on occasional panic attacks. Sound familiar? We're all aware of them, and the same hormones, perspiration, muscle tension, increased blood pressure and heartbeat, etc. surge within nanoseconds just as they did for cavemen. However, what we are not aware of is the demands they chronically place on our immune system in the form of damaging free radicals that destabilize normal cells. Common physical stressors include high fat diets, alcohol, food additives, smoking and radiation. Psychological stress and depression deplete our immune reserves, thus extracting a high price. The effect is cumulative unless we a) boost our immune system and b) look for places in life where we can "turn the volume down" on the number and kind of stressors that we live with. In most cases, we feel like it's easier said than done. A wise physician or psychotherapist, however, recognizes the interrelationship between a disease of the body and the lack of ease (or DIS-ease) in mind, emotions and spirit, and offers interdisciplinary solutions.

But coping with stress is not the exclusive property of medicine or psychotherapy. Besides healthy eating and nutritional supplements, life itself is filled with moments that calm down the stress response and replenish the immune system. Laughter, music, dance, vacations, the arts, close friendships and strong commitments are just a few ways to improve general psychological health and undo the damage to the immune system. Art therapy and occupational therapy have been applied successfully to mental problems for years. Yoga, martial arts such as Tai Chi and aerobic exercise are standard relaxation protocols in today's high stress world. Meditation lowers blood pressure and has improved lives for half a century in America. Thoughts, beliefs and attitudes can trigger a stress response, or prevent it. Pessimistic patients who give up the will to live often die prematurely, but optimistic patients who fight for life live longer. There are many things in life we can't control, but taking charge of our outlook is one thing each person can do.

I can attest to the fact that cancer support groups have great psychological value. When I lecture for these groups, I am encouraged to hear so many prostate cancer survivors proclaim that their post cancer life is better and more meaningful that their pre-cancer existence. Not only do many men feel better and function at a higher physical level than before they were diagnosed with their malignancy, but they enjoy life more. In fact, their body is often in better physical shape due to a dynamic change of life style and their satisfaction level is usually higher due to a new appreciation of life. Prayer is frequently a source of peace of mind that translates into a healthful and more positive future.

Hope from many natural sources

Nutrition and supplements are one aspect of promoting natural prevention and healing. Nature may have more surprises in store for us. Agents such as ozone and light, especially in the ultraviolet wavelength prove useful in treating disease through the blood system. A remedy proposed and validated by Dr. Majid Ali, Board Certified Surgeon and Board Certified Pathologist, is that of "dysoxygenosis and oxystatic therapy." In his 2004 book *Principles and Practice of Integrative Medicine*, Dr. Ali shows a lack of oxygen to cause disease states and demonstrates successful therapies that re-oxygenate the body emphasizing the use of hydrogen peroxide, ozone, oxygen and related substances that promote healing. Books have been written about the Rife energy cancer cure which may yet prove to be a viable resource for patients. The beneficial effect from strong magnetic fields on cancers deserves further evaluation. Dr. Larry Clapp's widely published book on prostate health *Prostate Health in 90 Days* has found many avid readers who have changed their lifestyles and improved their prostate disease. Immunotherapies are particularly important for patients who choose surgery, radiation or chemotherapies, since these modalities tend to depress the body's immune system. An interesting byproduct of the use of herbs, nutritional supplements and dietary changes for treatment of prostate cancer is the accompanying salutary health effects ameliorating heart disease, arthritis, BPH and prostatitis.

Finally, patients must have hope in the future of medicine to find new modalities for treating cancer. The non invasive and minimally invasive therapies I discuss in this book may still seem like science fiction to many specialists in the cancer field. My foundation, the Biofoundation for Angiogenesis Research and Development, is continually searching the frontiers of medical science to extract, document, refine and ultimately bring to patients the myriad of new possibilities for treating malignancies.

CHAPTER 11

CANCER SCREENING
PRO'S AND CON'S

Screening is hot business—hot for patients, because they get their fears resolved, and hot for providers, since their business is booming. Early detection of serious disease, such as coronary artery disease with electron beam computed tomography (EBCT-special CT scan showing calcification of the arteries to the heart) and screening for lung cancer with computed tomography (CT-scans) is commonplace and rising in popularity even though there is no proven reduction in mortality from these diseases by earlier discovery. Not only are these studies controversial, it is unclear at this time whether the potential benefits outweigh the risks. Common risks include unnecessary workups for false positive test results, excessive cost of "downstream" procedures, and false reassurance from false negative results. Risks from radiation and patient anxiety have not been fully assessed at this time, yet patients are paying out of pocket and physicians are referring for these exams. People pay for "peace of mind."

Knowledge versus preference

Merging doctor's knowledge (Informed Decision Making or IDM) with patient preference results in Shared Decision Making (SDM) in cancer care. A new model of medical decision-making has emerged that gives patients more responsibility for their own healthcare. The concept of SDM arose in the 1980's. This was partly due from pressures to develop evidence-based strategies for disease prevention and improve treatment outcomes. In cancer care, the idea gained credence with the increasing recognition of two facts:

- Numerous preventive and treatment options involve the potential for significant harm, while holding only limited promise for improvement.
- The fear of the risks and the desire for the benefits of any treatment are highly influenced by patients' personal values and preferences.

Over the years, clinicians have taken steps toward IDM by giving patients more information and broader perspective about the risks and benefits of treatments, but progress toward SDM has been slow. Many doctors have been reluctant to offer patients true choices that would let them determine for themselves whether or not one option better meets their values or allows them to reject a recommended course of treatment. Still, the trend is increasingly toward SDM.

As patients and clinicians embrace SDM, cancer patients will play a greater role in determining their treatment plan, including what screening or imaging studies will be performed. "It respects the concept that it's important when making treatment decisions to try to understand and incorporate patients' preferences and information they bring to the decision process," said Tim J. Whelan, BM, BCh, MSc, who moderated a panel discussion on SDM last October at the meeting of the American Society for Therapeutic Radiology and Oncology in Salt Lake City.

SDM requires asking hard questions, and physicians being willing to give full disclosure. Is it appropriate to offer an unproven screening test before it has been established through clinical trials? Is it wise to deny patients access to a screening that may give them relief from anxiety? Stress and anxiety are proven killers. Many cancers are not lethal. The vast majority of men would rather be told they have a prostate cancer—thus providing ease from fear—rather than live with uncertainty. Probably the worst effect of a false positive screening test is the undue worry about the effect of the disease on oneself and one's family. A secondary bad effect is the hassle and costs in terms of time and money of the unending follow up downstream tests to confirm the screening possibility.

What about the early detection of a disease for which there need be no treatment? In this case, ignorance is not only bliss, it is useful. What about the early detection of a problem for which there is no treatment? Perhaps ignorance cannot hurt in the long run. Early detection may not mean better care, either. In the case of removal of a small tumor detected by screening that leaves behind a larger parent malignancy that may have been found by standard medical care at a later interval, the patient has been disserved by earlier diagnosis. There is also a financial drain on the health care system when a screening turns up the need for additional testing and treatments. The deliverer of the screening may wish to educate the patient as to the unproven nature of the test and the potential risks associated with the procedure. For example, when patients learn the 97% accuracy of serious prostate cancer discovered by the combination of 3D PDS and MRI, many defer the biopsy which offers less than a 50-50 chance of confirmation in most patients. (Note that MRI-guided biopsies, while not yet the standard of care, do offer a remarkable degree of accuracy over the conventional TRUS biopsy. In addition, "fusion" software allows urologists with advanced technology such as the Artemis® device to merge their own ultrasound images with those of 3T MRI done by a radiologist for significant pinpointing of prostate tumors.) The possibility of a biopsy spreading the tumor is also foremost on the minds of most patients, even though their surgeons have down played this possibility. Many patients also rethink their treatment options when learning of the high rates of cancer recurrence following standard tumor therapy regimens. In fact, a study by Braddock in a 1999 issue of the *Journal of the American Medical Association* showed only 9% of patients met the criteria for IDM in the 3552 clinical decisions reviewed.

The 2007 *Journal of the American College of Radiology* defines 10 criteria for screening tests:

1. The disease has serious consequences
2. The screening population has a high prevalence of detectable preclinical phase
3. The test detects little pseudodisease (disease that would not become clinically significant)
   a) nonprogressive disease
   b) progressive, but not clinically significant

4. High accuracy in finding the detectable preclinical phase
5. Detecting disease before the critical point of clinical injury
6. Low morbidity
7. Test is affordable and available
8. Treatment exists
9. Treatment is more effective when applied before symptoms begin
10. Treatment is not too risky or toxic

The American College of Physicians has set forth a charter on the ethics of unproven screening tests that requires the physician to empower his or her patient to make informed decisions. IDM, informed decision making, includes the possible side effects of the tests, the accuracy and limitations inherent in the exam and the alternatives to the procedure including doing nothing. Screening options are also more complex with today's rapid technological advances. For colorectal cancer screening, patients may choose from the following menu: colonoscopy (entire colon), flexible sigmoidoscopy (lower colon), air-contrast barium enema (x ray study using air in an enema), fecal occult blood testing (detects blood in stool from bleeding tumor) and virtual colonoscopy (CT scans of inside of colon).

Patients must consider the risks and benefits of the PSA test for prostate cancer. Controversies still exist over the age to start mammograms and how often women should get Pap smears for cervical cancer. Patients, now more than ever, want to participate in their own care. Patients want a relationship with their physician based on mutual participation.

The widespread dissemination of accurate health information on the Internet and through dedicated cancer support groups gives patients the right to share their knowledge and informed opinions with those of their physicians. Indeed, much of what I have learned about alternative medicine comes from listening to the success stories of my patients. Remember that anecdotal evidence is valuable. When I hear of some strange medicament helping someone I put it in the back of my mind. If I hear ten men tell similar experiences, I shift this concept to the front of my mind and raise my antenna to listen for more details. When I hear a hundred men recount similar experiences from an herb I had no knowledge of, I find out more from the Internet and research the medical databases.

IDM occurs when the individual fully understands the nature and scope of the clinical service. That is, the expected outcome: likely consequences, including risks, limitations, benefits, alternatives and uncertainties. The patient must consider his preference as appropriate and feel he has fully participated in the decision making at a personally desirable level. IDM and SDM differ somewhat from legal informed consent. The legal medical consent is based upon the competence of both parties, full disclosure by the physician, understanding, voluntary agreement and lastly, consent by the patient. In contrast, IDM and SDM take into account the degree to which a patient may or may not choose to participate in a decision making process and focus on producing decisions consistent with patient' preferences and values.

Decision making is most important when there are several equal and valid tests available for the same medical problem. The patient must recognize that a test often involves more than a single encounter and the results frequently translate to a new medical journey upon which he must unwillingly travel. An article for radiologists in the *Journal of the American College of Radiology* in April 2005 asks diagnostic imagers who perform radiologic screening tests to learn from the lesson of the unproven PSA blood test. Citing evidence that there is no clear evidence that PSA screening reduces the mortality of prostate cancer, the American College of Physicians and the American Urological Association recommend that patients be informed of the known risks and potential benefits of PSA testing so they can make personal decisions about testing. The risks include further testing such as biopsy of the prostate from false positive results, unnecessary worry, and the side effects of common treatments (impotence and incontinence) when the natural course of the disease may not have affected a man's mortality.

One problem of testing is that up to one third of men who had PSA tests did not realize that was included in their testing series. This raises concern for the potential harm that may arise when men must cope with the consequences of a test they did not even know they had taken. The results of a simple test may lead to a cascade of future decisions about follow up testing and possibly various unpleasant treatments. While some argue the reassurance of a negative test results in a grateful patient, others note that the most aggressive prostate cancers do not make PSA and thus are not ruled out by a low or normal PSA level. Indeed, a European study of 2074 screening biopsies presented at the 100th AUA Meeting by Drs. W. Horninger and G. Bartsch confirmed that the percentage of high grade (Gleason greater than or equal to 7) cancers was substantial. In the PSA group of 1-2, there were 13% of high grade tumors; in the PSA group of 2-3, there were 22% of high grade cancers, and, in the PSA group of 3-4, there were 22% of high grade cancers.

Dr. Klotz's article on active surveillance in Chapter 7 also invites discussion of current screening concepts for prostate cancer. He notes, "If all American men between 50-70 with PSA>2.5 had a biopsy…775,000 cases of cancer would be found…which is 25 times (2500% higher) than the 30,350 men expected to die of PC per year in the US." He quotes the 2004 *Canadian Cancer Journal* article by Jemal demonstrating the lifetime risk of dying from prostate cancer remaining at less than 3%. His own phase III study is showing that aggressive treatment of PC improves survival for 1 out of every 100 patients. He does not take into consideration the problem of interval cancers. As I stated in the 2006 *JFR* meeting, interval tumors are highly aggressive and occur within 6 months. This is why our group performs screening sonography of the breast and prostate at half yearly intervals. Our two year study showed about 5% of men developed high grade prostate tumors every 6 months which was clearly demonstrable by 3D PDS and confirmed by DCE-MRI.

Studies presented at the May 2005 New York Roentgen Society Annual Meeting in New York showed that imaging with MRI and ultrasound detects cancers better than biopsy alone and should be used to guide biopsies for greater accuracy. Dr. Hedvig Hricak, Director of Radiology at Memorial Sloan Kettering Cancer Center, noted up to 80% of tumors were missed by standard (non image guided) biopsies. In fact, the study also showed that of the successful biopsies, 48% were inaccurately read when compared to the postoperative specimen carefully examined in the pathology department. (The full text of the presentation is appended to the end of the book). Dr. Daniel Kopans, Professor of Radiology at Harvard Medical School, mentioned in his 2005 talk at the New York Cancer Society that current methods were not successful in predicting metastatic potential of cancers and suggested that blood flow analyzed by ultrasound Doppler imaging would be helpful.

I implemented an IDM and SDM system in my office at the beginning of 2004. My patients are seated in front a computer and view a presentation of my tests and possible treatments with limitations and side effects so they can make their independent decision. During my testing, I show my patient exactly what I am seeing on a large overhead screen and especially highlight areas of concern and explain their nature. After my testing results are explained to my patient, I sit with him (and wife/partner, if available) and we make shared decisions. I give my patients a preliminary report to read. I then go over what they understood with their family, if present, and what they choose to do for treatment. I also hand them a copy of their final report, a set of ultrasound images on a compact disc and a written sheet of paper listing all the possible treatments, with their side effects, including phone numbers of other specialists to whom they may speak directly.

Through the Biofoundation for Angiogenesis R&D, I have developed relationships with the worldwide leaders in many areas of prostate medicine. Most have agreed to work together as a team to advance the state of prostate cancer treatment and personally advise patients courageous enough to consider alternative and probable future FDA approved treatments. These dedicated and busy physicians will, to make further breakthroughs in medicine, give of their time to confer with and support men trying to make a better life by taking a chance on promising new technologies. To paraphrase Mother Teresa, do a little good with a lot of love and eventually the world will be a better place. Tony Cointreau, who worked with Mother Teresa in India and became her trusted biographer, was presented as the 2005 Humanitarian Award winner in New York City. On the celebrity-packed stage, he said: "The simple truth, starting with a whisper, kindled by hope, reinforced by courage, emboldened by commitment and strengthened by knowledge will evolve, triumph and impact the world like a comet."

I ask my patients, if they so wish, to consult their hearts, their minds, their family, their friends, their physicians and spiritual advisors and call me in a week or so to refine their decisions with me. Results by Dr. A. Wolf in the 1996 *Archives of Internal Medicine* noted that decision aids improved knowledge, decreased interest in PSA screening and increased interest and participation in the decision making process. An ethical approach to unproven screening tests being developed suggests that health care providers fulfill the five components of informed consent with their patients:

1. Assess a patient's competence to make a decision
2. Disclose the key facts
3. Make sure the patient understands by asking the patient what he heard
4. Make sure the patient can make a voluntary decision
5. Make sure the patient is able to give consent

An open ended question such as: "Tell me in your own words how you arrived at your decision, the risks and benefits you see, and the options you are considering," is a sentence I find helpful with my patients to establish and review their decision process. One problem in discussing options is the divide between the complex nature of medicine and the personal nature of and individual patient needs. In addition to asking men what their personal considerations are, I inform them of facts that previous patients have told me about quality of life issues that were not apparent until after the tests and treatments were undertaken, such as: "After HIFU occasionally I would find fragments of my prostate in the urine;" "After hormones my hip fractured;" "After antioxidants I lost 15 pounds;" "On plant hormones my skin got better and my wife (and my mistress) started stealing my pills," etc. I then tailor my responses to individual concerns. For example, complaints I have heard about the post HIFU cancer treatment experience have included the need for a catheter to be worn in the penis for a few weeks. While most men accepted this as a necessary evil, one of my patients challenged me, saying he would risk the procedure without a catheter or he would not be treated at all. I discussed this option with my team and we came up with the alternative of placing a catheter through a tiny abdominal incision into the bladder (called a "suprapubic catheter") instead of inside the penis. This worked so well on this patient that it has now become the standard of post treatment HIFU care, and actually improved the postoperative course by reducing the time for urination to return to normal on all patients and contributing greatly to patient comfort at the same time. According to the ethics guidelines of the American College of Radiology, since many patients are referred to me directly by friends and family, and not by other physicians, I am obligated to inform them of the risks, benefits and limitations of my testing. I request my patients and potential referring physicians look at my website **www. bardcancercenter.com** before and after they see me to be maximally informed and make any suggestions that may improve the informational content. I mention that my equipment is specifically calibrated to detect the 3% of cancer that is lethal and may not always detect some of the remaining 97% that is not overtly lethal and can be managed conservatively. I highlight studies from international medical centers showing that the 3D PDS is 95% accurate in detecting Gleason 7 or higher, may show seminal vesicle invasion and usually discerns extracapsular spread on the 3-D reconstruction and analysis of the 800 to 1400 images that are captured as a reference data set in the computer and studied on a radiologic 4-D workstation. When indicated by high suspicion of spread outside the capsule, I obtain an MRI that shows adjacent lymph nodes and metastases to bones and the adjacent seminal vesicles. The MRI is much more sensitive in this regard than the CT scan and has no radiation. The new computer-aided MRI showing abnormal blood vessels combined with the 3D PDS has added greatly to the follow up of treated tumors. If suspicious lymph nodes are detected, the new *Combidex* MRI performed in Europe shows if the tumor has spread to the nodes, and which nodes are involved. The combination of DCE-MRI and 3D PDS is 97 % accurate in detecting significant cancers. Of greatest importance is the ability to demonstrate the response of a vascular tumor to therapy within a short period of time that provides patients with a milestone marker with which to better guide their treatment plan and follow up periodically on the chosen therapy.

CHAPTER 12

AN OPEN MIND IS
YOUR BEST FRIEND

Primum non nocere. "First, Do No Harm."
—From the physician's sacred Hippocratic Oath

This chapter is designed to give the reader a sense of how to use this book's information in his personal life. Some readers are extremely knowledgeable about cancer and cancer treatments; and for other patients, this book is the first information they have been able to read to find out more about cancer options. This time in a cancer patient's life is tremendously frightening as well as bewildering for him. In order for the book to be useful and valuable, I invite the reader to think about how the material presented could make a difference in addressing his particular personal health problems or perhaps, the health problems of a loved one.

Study cancer with an open mind. Search for new ideas, and compare them with what physicians and cancer societies promote as "accepted" facts. Will the comparison reinforce existing ideas, beliefs and values—or will it open a world of enlightenment? It is human nature to want to be right; subconsciously, one gathers evidence to support preconceived ideas and turn opinions into facts. Gleaning value from this book requires an inquisitive nature and a thirst for knowledge.

When people learn, they often learn through an unconscious filter. For example, if a person puts on a pair of yellow sunglasses, everything would appear yellow. However, if the person leaves them on for a week, things wouldn't appear yellow, they would appear normal. This is called the "already-always" way of learning, and for many readers it applies to the way they approach this book.

Take this question: What does everyone know about teen-agers? A man thinks, "That's the way my teenagers are." He simply accepts preconceived ideas. A more powerful way of reading this book is for an individual to embrace an open mind. Read and digest the contents, but try it without the usual filter, whatever it may be.

A personal example of the "already-always" thinking is the day my car was towed away. I had parked legally in front of my office on East 60th street in the early evening. When I stepped out, I saw a police tow truck towing my car down the block. I had apparently failed to see a small paper sign warning of a movie shooting sequence on the street and allowing no parking during that time period. At any rate, as I saw the official tow truck cross over Park Avenue with my vehicle dangling in the back, I knew that I would have to recover my car later from the tow pound by the Hudson River piers on the west side of town. I knew it would take a few hours to tag the car in the system before I could recover it. I called up at midnight, and the car was not in the pound. "Call back later," said the officer. By 2:00 A.M. the car had not yet been logged into the data base. I decided to wait until the next day. Many calls throughout the day netted me no information of the whereabouts of my car. I finally spoke with the desk sergeant and told him from where my car had been removed. He checked with the temporary towing department, and informed me that my car had been moved a block and a half west of my original parking spot. Even worse was the realization that I had walked past it several times that day in broad daylight and not recognized it! Obviously, I "knew" it had been towed away to where I expected. How many people will read this book and miss its value because of their (or their doctors' or the "experts'") assumptions about where today's world of prostate cancer is "parked"?

It could be said that health education is additive—where an individual studies and learns, and the more he puts in, the more he gets out—and the results may be surprising and unexpected. When scientists work (and I am a scientist), they dwell in a problem, dwell in an issue, or dwell in a specific area to finally make a breakthrough. They carefully examine all facets of the problem to find a reasonable solution. They have done all the preparation, obtained all the available information, and keep bumping up against questions and struggling against answers and brainstorming for solutions; finally, "AHA!" An epiphany occurs! It is very much like turning a light on in a dark room. They suddenly see something they have never seen before. It all comes together—something is made possible that was never possible before. That's the kind of awakening I wish for the reader to experience from this book.

One specific tool often underused is "listening" to your doctor. Men don't want to hear bad news, yet that is the access to power. In written Chinese, the word for "crisis" is made up of two parts: one represents danger, the other opportunity. Your health problem is your health opportunity, and you need information to take charge of the situation. Verify with your physician what you heard by repeating it back and asking for a written report. I speak with my patients initially, then hand them a written report and ask them to read it and speak with me again. If you are unclear, call back the same day or as soon as possible to have your questions answered. Remember that there are no stupid questions. This is your health! No, this is your life at stake! Do not ask for certainty, but get clarity about available options and side effects.

Here's a personal example of "incomplete" listening. The Germans have a popular phrase for this kind of discontinuous communication: *Sie reden einander vorbei*, meaning "they speak past one another." I believe in aerobic exercise for health and I take weekly ballroom dancing lessons. There is a big sign in the dance studio: I KNOW YOU HEARD WHAT I SAID, BUT WHAT YOU THINK I TOLD YOU IS NOT WHAT I MEANT YOU TO DO. I was learning a standard dance step called the cross body lead. The man steps back and guides his partner past him across his body. The man's body moves 90 degrees away from the woman thus opening a door like a swinging gate, allowing the woman to dance straight ahead through the opening he has just created. Instead, I moved back at a 45 degree angle and when it didn't work, I was frustrated. I told my instructor I had followed the directions to the letter. When the video was replayed, I was astounded that my mind told me my body was acting according to the given instructions even though my body was moving in a direction different from my strict intentions. I now judge the effectiveness of communication by what people do rather than what they say they understand.

This analogy is applicable to my patients. I follow up and verify what happens clinically at 3 to 6 month intervals. Most failures stem from noncompliance of therapeutic instructions—specifically, some men stop treatment when they feel better, some stop to try other regimens, some substitute impure foreign made antioxidants for American made products, some reduce the effectiveness by taking other pills and herbs that neutralize the treatment regimen, etc.

Shifting the limits or paradigms in which a person operates

What is a paradigm? Essentially a paradigm defines the limits of the way each person perceives life around him or the way he defines his world. It's a pattern or mold that each man follows. It is a precise learned way of thinking. It is sort of a background phenomenon—a way of thinking or knowing something. An American, for example, has certain ways of perceiving his "Americanism" that are obvious to him, but when he goes to another culture, people think very differently about those same things because of their own paradigms that mold their thinking about "Americanism."

We find daily examples of people limited by their paradigms, be they simple or profound. I was lecturing at the Mayo Clinic division in Scottsdale, Arizona in 1994, I had occasion to be in a fabric store in nearby Phoenix. I saw a pretty umbrella in a stand by the door. When I asked how much it was, they said: "It's not for sale. We're in the desert. Here umbrellas are used only for decoration." If the salesperson could have shifted out of the idea that umbrellas are only for rain, he could have advertised and sold them for protection from the sun, like the delightful parasols that Asian women use to protect their skin. This would have been utilizing possibilities by thinking outside the box.

In shifting away from old ideas and assumptions, a person can create whole new possibilities for moving life forward—and break through to accept new, dynamic ideas. It's not merely about trying out a different solution. It's that the paradigm entirely changes.

Centuries ago, people used to think evil spirits caused disease, and the methods of curing disease ranged from drilling holes in heads to let out the evil spirits, to bleeding patients. Next, germs and bacteria were discovered. That discovery completely altered the entire field of medicine and the possibilities of how to diagnose and treat disease.

Another way to exemplify what I mean by operating outside the current paradigm is exemplified by the 9 dots puzzle below. Thinking outside the box is a valuable way to stretch the imagination. The object in solving this game is to connect all 9 dots without removing the pencil from the paper and using a continuous and uninterrupted line.

9 DOTS PUZZLE

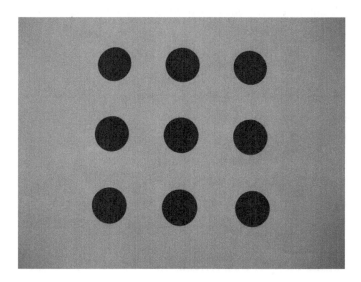

To solve the puzzle, one must connect all 9 dots by using four straight connected lines. The lines must be continuous. Most people try to solve this inside the box because that's the normal paradigm in which most people think. But, when one goes outside of the box, whole new solutions are possible. Simply extending line 1 past the last dot opens up a previously unpredictable possibility.

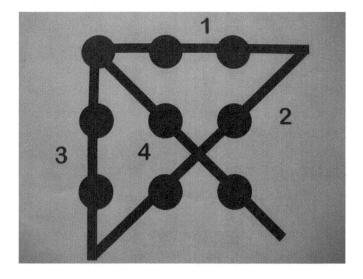

Another powerful example is: centuries ago in Western Europe, the academics, rulers and common people knew the world was flat. Exploration was out of the question! Sailors rarely ventured beyond a certain distance from the coast, and only along established routes. It's not that they didn't have the technology for exploration, or the tools for navigating. A flat world was the only paradigm available at the time, and everyone operated consistent with this idea, such as not sailing over the horizon. When the world was demonstrated to be round, whole new possibilities become available.

When fleas are placed in a jar with a lid cover, the fleas will jump until they hit the lid. After the lid is removed they still only jump as high as the lid. That limit becomes the extent of their paradigm even though, in actuality, far more room to jump is available. Human beings, including physicians, are sometimes similar to fleas. For example, when some people express themselves too freely, they get hurt. If this happens repetitively, they withdraw to protect themselves. Because they are vulnerable to pain, they give themselves invisible limits. Unfortunately, people live in safe and comfortable mindsets where life is limited but "bearable." Physicians, too, are afraid to try new treatments and are understandably satisfied with their current routines. Patients may consider jumping out of the jar when their current options do not look promising. The modern equivalent is to open a computer and search on Google.

The book provides the ability to identify the paradigms from which the reader is thinking. A person might not even be cognizant of the trap or limited situation his mind is in. Here the reader has access to invent new paradigms for himself that give him a far broader range of possibilities. Try asking: What are the imaginary boxes I'm living confined in? What treatments are available that I'm not even aware of? If I wait, will there be new and better therapies next year? When a patient sees new possibilities, he regains hope. He perceives something that he hasn't been able to perceive before. He realizes a wide variety of therapies that treat cancer and manage disease are now available to choose at his doorstep. Please read of the inspirational health crusade undertaken by one of my Australian patients in his email to a prostate cancer alternative group displayed as follows:

2005 e-mail letter from Australia:

i was dxd with pc in 1996 at age 45 and was almost bullied into a RP…however i told the urologist (one of the top ones in sydney at st vincents hospital) that he had no idea what he was doing to all these young men and i proceeded to give him the statistics…in the years to come he actually told me that he would never have one himself!!!)…

i was fortunate to have the resources to abandon my business life for a time and travel the world looking for a cure…my path led me to beijing, china (i was chairman of a company building thousands of houses for the government) where i was "inspected" by the head of the cancer hospital and then by deng's personal physician, and then another expert who travelled 30 hours from Mongolia…they all said the same thing… my body was out of balance with too much "yang"…the chinese believe that the body can only be in a state of "disease" if the yin/yang balance is disturbed and this in turn causes a blockage of "chi" or energy, prana, electrical current or whatever you call it… they also believe that the body has yin and yang organs..the yin organs being the "wet" ones, liver, kidneys, pancreas, digestive system and the yang organs,"dry" and the heart, brain and lungs…the yin organs are the ones that control and monitor the immune system and cancer is an autoimmune disease so the key is to fix the immune system.

yang organs are boosted by adrenaline (fight or flight syndrome which inflicts the western world and is part of our way of life, constantly dribbling the dreaded chemicals whenever the phone rings) and the yin organs are boosted by balance and harmony (meditation, prayer, quiet etc)…it all made sense to me so after 3 weeks a treatment by a chi master i returned home feeling amazing.

i cleaned out my body with a 10 day fast, and a colema regime based on bernard jensen's philosophy, took up meditation again (i was a TM meditator 20 years earlier so was easy to fall right back in) and consumed vast amounts of stinking chinese herbs that i had brought home …my psa started to fall.

i read a lot of books by deepak chopra and his mind/body connection made a lot of sense…i had been a property developer for 20 years with lots of staff, debt and with an A type personality that was constantly pushing life's boundaries…(its interesting to note that PC is a disease of mostly A type personalities…there is 2.5 times the amount of PC in the US congress than the general population… all A types, bad diet, travel and constant fight or flight syndrome.) so i thought deepak was my man…i took a plane to san diego to meet and greet him… we became friends and i travelled to india with him constantly absorbing his healing message which is deeply reflective of the chinese, indian philosophy based around the mind/ body relationship and life balance, meditation etc….one of the first things deepak said to me was "andrew, what is causing this disease…look at your life and tell me"…i knew so very soon after this i got a divorce and set out with a new partner …my marriage was toxic and i knew deep down that it was making me ill.

around this stage i became aware of larry clapp and was amazed how close his philosophy and healing path was to the one i had developed for myself…i also became aware of sophie chen and pc-spes so i jumped on that chat group and for 5 years took her concoction…the results of all this was great with my psa normal at about 2, my life rearranged and i was meeting a great bunch of guys through the site…of course all this went when the discovery was made that tiny amounts of prescription drugs (DES) was in the purported herbal capsules and greedy men started to sue and reported the company, botaniclabs, to the authorities…thus one of the best PC mixtures was banned and to this date no one has been able to replicate the formula…although Dr DONBACH is having success with his similar formula.

I have an annual checkup with my very clever friend, dr robert bard in new york and in february he declared me cancer free although my last psa test was about 6…he says to ignore this and stop having it done.

i am fit and well and have sired another child recently (i now have 4), i am back building a few buildings but gently and without the extreme passion of days gone…i ran into the urologist (who wanted to operate in 1996 and told me i would be dead in three years if i didnt pay heed) at a party last xmas…he said he was still doing biopsies and RPs but really didn't believe they worked (what a dangerous path this guy is travelling…and i read in a sydney paper that he had bought a $6 million dollar house, so business must be good at $10,000 a pop) and he was now asking his patients to make up their own minds about the type of treatment path they chose rather than trying to bully them as he had done me.

so guys even though none of us asked to join this club we are all in it and helping each other…i believe my diagnosis has been a great gift in that it has lead me to all sorts of changes and new friends and situations…my "gods" have so far been very kind.

love and good health.

AR [name withheld]

As I was writing this chapter, a physician in our professional complex came in for an x-ray of his nose. He had injured his nose during a tennis match that morning. After I read the x-rays that suggested a fracture rather than confirmed one, I asked myself if there was a better way to look at the tiny bones in the nasal area. I had just read an article about x-rays missing 90% of rib fractures. X-rays of curved bones do not see all the borders. I knew from performing sonograms of the rotator cuff in the shoulder that I could detect fractures of the humerus better than the routine x-rays. I had also diagnosed wrist dislocations and rib fractures with regular sonogram techniques for years. However, as Chief of Radiology in 1980 at Manhattan's Eye and Ear Hospital, I knew how difficult fractures of the nose were to diagnose—even with dedicated x-ray equipment.

I wondered if I could perform a 3-D scan on the injured area. The 3-D probe for the "small parts" of the body is 4 cm or 2 inches wide and is usually used for breast or thyroid imaging. I thought of mustard on a hot dog in a bun. My idea was to let the hot dog be the nose and allow the bun be a container that holds a large quantity of ultrasound "gel" or coupling agent (mustard, in the analogy) in which the large probe face could rest. Then, I placed surgical tape to make receptacle for the gel around the nose sparing the nostrils, filled the area to the top with coupling material and obtained a beautiful 3-D picture of the nasal bones showing definite but non-displaced fractures on both sides.

Human beings are designed to resist or change things that are unwanted, unpleasant or irritating to them. Human beings, mostly men, are designed to react in anger and frustration when our intention is interrupted. That's just the way our human "machinery" works, so to speak. When the reader comprehends the actual "design mechanism" in cancer, he will have a new power over the outcome and be able to control the results and better endure the process. You can't change the fact that you have cancer and complaining certainly will not make any difference. You can, however, make promises and requests. Promises such as: I will drink green tea and alter my diet, I will engage in aerobic exercises, I will search the internet for new treatments, etc. Requests such as: I will ask men about successful treatments, I will find support groups, I will tell my family and friends to assist me in lifestyle changes, I will query cancer foundations, etc.

An example that is common in my practice is erectile dysfunction, (ED). The very thought of a prostate problem robs men of libido. The threat of prostate surgery produces fear and stress which often leads to impotence. While this can't be changed, the option of non-invasive therapies or minimally invasive treatments improves men's sexual performance. Additionally, drugs such as Cialis and Viagra permit satisfactory sex lives when undergoing the various hormone castration protocols. The new and effective health alternatives render current problems less frustrating.

Creating a team

Teamwork forwards events more effectively and frequently faster. I consider my patients as part of my team. Men and often, their wives, forward successful outcomes to my attention as well as negative treatment side effects. For example, women with breast cancer have reported control of their tumor by injections of *botulinum neurotoxin a or b* (Botox or Myobloc) in and around the abnormal growth. No side effects have been described from this. One of my patients heard about this and decided to try this on his recurrent prostate cancer. He had radiation for Gleason 9 disease and had a recurrence 10 months later. This was treated with HIFU (high intensity focused ultrasound) but the tumor recurred again. In despair, his recurrence was injected with neurotoxin in Europe resulting in stabilization for six months. At his half year follow up, the treated area was inactive but a new tumor occurred on the opposite side. He had repeat HIFU therapy and both sides were stable at his 1-year follow up. Two years later boney metastases occurred and he departed this world, as we all must, but not without a "fight." In the end, he had his pride to comfort him. He was a champion, not a victim, and that had earned him several more unexpected years of life.

One reason to build a health care team is to reduce human error. Errors result from the natural physiological and psychological limitations of human beings. Sources of error commonly include fatigue, workload, mental overload, poor interpersonal communications, imperfect information processing and flawed decision making. Teamwork can help overcome all of these.

Team creation is necessary since no one person can do it all in today's complex world. Each team member must have an area of personal responsibility. For example, the physician provides treatment, the patient follows a planned therapy, the wife or nurse makes sure the patient keeps his commitment to health, family members offer support, etc. The more members in a team, the greater the chance of catching and correcting any errors. On a practical note, the presence of an effective team enhances communication and reduces stress through overall better performance. Going one better, the presence of a great team offers the joy of connectedness, and the gift of being able to give back in unexpected ways.

Effective use of a team requires an invitation to participate in your care. One must encourage team members to provide information, express their concerns and speak up when necessary. The patient must show respect for all the team and put his ego below the good intentions of the support group. Imaging saying, "Botox is for women," and turning off any future possibility that may derive from an open mind. The industrialist, Henry Ford put teamwork this way "Coming together is a beginning. Keeping together is progress. Working together is success."

An important function of the team is to recognize adverse situations by looking for red flags or warning signs. The usual indicators of adversity are: conflicting information, preoccupation, poor communication and departure from usual practice. At the first sign of adversity, actively seek the help and comfort of others. Let us say the physician has had a rough day and is both stressed and fatigued. He may be curt or distracted or both. You may hear: "This is an aggressive tumor" at the beginning of the visit and "Let me see you in six months" and the end of the consultation. Signs of poor doctor communication include talking too much and/ or not listening to you. Signs of poor patient communication include obsessing over unimportant test results (such as PSA) and thinking you understand fully what is being said. As the patient, you have the right to demand specific measurable performance from each member of your health team. Remember, the design of the team is to assist you in making the best health care decisions possible. So keep your team "machinery" well oiled and you will have a smoother ride through your illness. Perhaps your support group is negative and continually warns you that every cancer is deadly and the treatments are worse than dying. If you can't empower them with a presentation of up to date facts, take action and change support groups. It is your responsibility to make your life better. Realize that there are no victimizers, only willing victims. Your health is ultimately in your hands and your doctor is part of your health team. Men who take charge of their lives more often prevail against prostate cancer.

A mission for a team to develop new treatments might look like this: Ask a PC survivor to grow a designated herb in a garden, take it for half a year and report what happens to an assigned person. Then ask him to request two other men to do the same with different plants and have each of the two new participants to enroll another two men to follow suit. It has been estimated 25% of the plant botanical varieties have been identified to date. Countless potential herbal sources are available to be studied. This scenario could create a team of 100,000 men and hundreds of new medical treatments within one year. How would you like to multiply your chances for beating cancer and living a fuller life? The hardest part of progress is to take a first step. Make it a small one, if you must, but start immediately. If it doesn't work out, start again. You've already taken the step of reading this book—now take another, then another, until you are striding forward knowing you have empowered yourself. Action takes the sting out of defeat, buffers the misery of disease and moves us forward out of despair into the fullness of life. As the French say, *"A votre santé."* To your health!

EPILOGUE

I thank each and every person who reads this book for allowing me to share my experience and knowledge. It is my hope that in addition to having provided established facts, persuasive logic, and intelligent examples, I have also provided hope and encouragement to men who are either concerned that they are at risk for prostate cancer, or have already been diagnosed. The greatest help I can offer is to empower men to understand their disease, embrace imaging as a necessary step before rushing into a biopsy, explore all treatment options, and turn to all personal and informational resources in making a decision. If I have been successful in doing so, then I have more than met my goals in writing this book.

ACKNOWLEDGMENTS

I thank Loreto Bard, Executive Director of the Biofoundation for Angiogenesis Research and Development, for her assistance in coordinating international multidisciplinary medical exchanges that advanced the concepts developed in this book. I wish to thank Drs. Duke Bahn, Stanley Brosman, Arthur Lurvey, Mark Scholz and Charles Myers (Prostate Cancer Research Institute); Drs. Giuseppe Brisinda, Federica Cadeddu and Giorgio Maria (the Catholic University Hospital in Rome, Italy); Drs. Thayne Larson, Benjamin Larson and Lance Mynderse (the Mayo Clinic Foundation); Dr.Francoise Giuliano (the Academic Hospital of Bicetre); Drs. Susan Keay and John Warren (The Prostatitis Foundation); Drs. Richard Stock, Lincoln Pao, Michael Zelefsky, Shalom Kalnicki (NY Roentgen Society); Drs. Guy Frija, Olivier Helenon, J-F Moreau and J-M Correas (Societe Francaise de Radiologie); Drs. J-L Sauvain, R Palasac and P. Palasac (the Paul Morel Hospital, Vesoul, France); Drs. Roberto Passariello and Vito Cantisani (Istituto Radiologia, Policlinico Umberto I, Rome, Italy); Drs. Bertrand Dufour, N. Thiounn, and Y. Chretien (Groupe Hospitalier Necker-Enfants Malades, Paris, France); Dr. David Cosgrove and Sir Richard Sykes (Imperial College of Medicine, London, England); Drs. William DeWolf, Edward Messing, Louis Denis, Eric Rovner, Ernest Sosa, Alexis Te, Michael Manyak, Michael Marberger, Joseph Smith, Jr, Harris Nagler, J. Fracchia, Peter Scardino, M. Droller, P. Schlegel, S. Kaplan, H. Lepor, M. Grasso, N. Romas, A. Melman, I. Grunberger, R. Macchia,

M. Choudhury, Victor Nitti and Patrick Walsh (American Urological Association); Drs. Marvin Rotman and Howard Hochster (New York Cancer Society); Dr. Jelle Barentsz, president of the International Cancer Imaging Society, for developing lymph node detection technology and disseminating awareness throughout the medical profession. Special thanks to Drs. Catherine Roy, Francois Cornud, Olivier Helenon, Peter Scardino, Michael Schachter, Ralph Moss, Ethan Halpern and Majid Ali whose books have provided new hope for cancer victims and further advanced medical knowledge. Thanks to Dr. Chris Renna, for his pioneering use of antioxidants.

LOST CURES FROM LOST CIVILIZATIONS

A good business consultant will tell you the first rule is to keep the clientele you have because someone else will be trying to win them over. A better consultant will ask to see what is missing in your endeavors. But successful medical treatments long lost over the centuries have obviously not kept their "clientele." They could use a 21st century investigating agent to represent their interests in recovering what worked in the past and has been forgotten in modern memory.

For example, cave paintings indicate that our remote ancestors used rose petals to treat disease. The use of this flower, used today to symbolize various kinds of love, continued into ancient recorded history in many cultures—perhaps symbolizing a love and appreciation for physical wellness on many levels. Chinese medicine recommends rose petal extract for regulating vital energy (qi) for strengthening blood circulation, purifying the liver and for alleviating joint pains. Rose petal essential oils were used as a dermal rehydrator to beautify the skin by the ancient Egyptians. In Roman times people treated breast diseases, skin conditions and even wound infections with orally ingested preparations.

The particular rose species *Rosa gallica* is gaining renewed respect in our contemporary world. The high concentration of anthocyanins in the petals are known for their ability to strengthen the vascular system, prevent blood platelet stickiness (blood clots) and also have powerful antioxidant, antibacterial and anti-inflammatory activity. Research has shown that an extract from *Rosa gallica* strikingly increases the effectiveness of several antibiotics against methicillin-resistant Staphylococcus aureus. Two active compounds from the extract have been identified as tellimagrandin I and rugosin B. Other studies have demonstrated strong activity of *Rosa gallica* extract against strains of Candida albicans isolated from overtreatment with antibiotics. Additionally, the effect of an anthocyanin preparation isolated from the flower petals of *Rosa gallica* demonstrated strong effects of Rosa extracts against abnormal cells. A five year research study by the Biofoundation for Angiogenesis Research preceded the development of the chemical constituents of the ProRose+ formulation. Scientific evaluation has shown the antioxidant effect to be ten times more powerful than green tea preparations and resveratrol formulations. Collagen regeneration has been observed clinically and documented with high resolution sonograms and special laser exams called optical coherent tomography (OCT). Improved blood flow to hair follicles has been demonstrated with vascular imaging technologies. The 2012 World Antiaging Conference showed poor dermal penetration of creams but good tissue regeneration with internal absorption of orally taken antioxidants.

We know many hidden cures are yet to be discovered in the primitive South American jungles, teeming Brazilian rain forests, vast stretches of Australia or arid deserts of Africa. But what has already been discovered and lost in the turmoils of history? One such person, a descendant of my wife, Loreto, to whom this book is dedicated, had a great, great grandfather, James Aquinas Ried, born in 1810. Tracing his earlier history revealed an extraordinary path of events through lost civilizations and promising medical discoveries. Dr. Ried was born in southern Germany, in Bavaria near Regensburg, in Castle Strahlfels. He went to the Scottish school for undergraduate work and the Royal University of Munich where in 1830 he obtained a Doctorate of Philosophy. He later emigrated to England and met the Duke of Wellington, who championed his advanced surgical training at the Royal College of Surgeons, in London. His character, as memorialized in his poetry and non medical prose, showed a determination to challenge existing political ideas and medical dogma.

With the help of the Duke of Wellington, he became a military physician for the British Government who posted him with the 96th Regiment in the northern province of Norfork 1, Australia for seven years. There he learned more about herbal treatments while visiting the aboriginal tribesmen and treating them on his long journeys by horseback. As the head physician of the military presidio, he used local medicaments to treat the population of the British garrison with success.

He later moved to Chile where he also taught European medicine to the local physicians. His curiosity (and courage) allowed him to meet with the fierce Mapuche Indians of the Chilean outback. These savages were known to strip the skin off of living men before eating them. However, the Indians had unique forms of medicine derived from local plants and trees which prevented certain diseases. He was also trained as a pharmacist and made extracts from collected varieties of certain flora which were used effectively as therapeutic agents. There exists in this area a massive machine press to extract ingredients from plants, possible invented by him. Remember, in those days you concocted your own plant remedies.

Eventually, he settled his life in Valparaiso, Chile (a prominent seaport near Santiago). While there he founded the German Hospital which remains today one of the country's leading medical institutions. Although he was a prolific writer and investigator, much of his work and research were destroyed during the Spanish naval bombardment of Valparaiso in 1866 (shortly before he died in 1869) and after following the great earthquake of 1906.

Loreto and I are trying to recreate the herbal formulations that a man of this caliber would have collected by searching the historical records in Australia, Germany, England and Chile. He was a "man for all seasons" having written the first Opera in the Spanish language (*TELESFORA ISMELDA IL GRANATIERE)*, authored a book in German: LEBENSBILD EINES DEUTSCHEN IN CHILE, pioneered the use of music as an adjunct to healing and created the first FIRE DEPARTMENT in the community of Valparaiso. This is yet another example that initiating the first step on a trail may lead one around the world to discover lost medical cures of a physician who created and brought western medicine to two continents. Today, the country of Peru is discovering many herbal varieties with significant healing powers never before revealed to the world. The Biofoundation for Angiogenesis is working with the Peruvian ambassador, Maria Teresa Merino de Hart, to catalogue and test these potential cures.

TESTIMONIALS

April 18, 2013 – Dr. Bob Waters

I am a 64-year old Medical doctor who trained in genetics and molecular biology prior to medical school. After a two-year surgical internship and orthopedic residency, I left to do general practice. I soon began basing my practice on nutrition and lifestyle. I learned in life that nutrition and lifestyle were the keys to health. I ate real, unprocessed foods, stayed lean and took nutritional supplements from age 30. It came as a big surprise when a routine life insurance physical at age 59 uncovered a prostate specific antigen (PSA) level of 3.8. I hadn't done one on myself for 15 years when it was under 1.0. I immediately repeated the PSA and it was 3.2. I reasoned that I couldn't have cancer because of my health practices and excellent family history.

I immediately repeated the PSA with a Free PSA measurement. This resulted in a PSA of 2.8 with a percent Free PSA of 14% indicating an increased probability of cancer. I was a little alarmed at this point but still figured I couldn't have cancer.

I had no urinary tract symptoms. Reasoning that I must have age-associated prostatic hypertrophy or a mild infection, I undertook a program of oral herbal formulas and other supplements including saw palmetto, pygeum, nettle extract, bee pollen, zinc, selenium, boron and stepped up my curcumin, siliphos, bioflavinoids, and other anti-cancer herbals. I did not consult a physician. Over the next two years my PSA ranged from 2.8 to 4.1.

In late 2010 and early 2011, I went through tremendous stress and felt progressively more ill—fatigue, deep aches in my long bones, muscle twitching, depression, night sweats and emotional swings. My PSA was 4.5 despite all I did, including high doses of intravenous vitamin C, Alpha lipoic acid, and a variety of antioxidants and other nutrients. My serum calcium had been high for some years, but I attributed this to my elevated albumin, which carries calcium in the bloodstream. Had I calculated the real calcium it would have revealed a serious increased level.

In the summer of 2011 I learned I had an elevated parathyroid hormone level and also very high urine calcium. The diagnosis of Primary Hyperparathyroidsm (PHP) was established and surgery was planned. This is important because men with PHP have threefold increase in prostate cancer presumably due to calcific deposits, which cause chronic inflammation of the gland.

I wanted to avoid biopsy of my prostate gland because of the possibility of needle track spreading of cancer so I sought other noninvasive tests. I found that a urine test, PCA-3 was more specific than PSA for prostate cancer (about 75% accurate). It measures a non-folded RNA fragment preferentially made by prostate cancer cells vs. normal cells. I had a rectal exam, which is needed prior to the test urine collection. My PCA-3 level was 177 with a reference range of less than 35. Now I was fairly sure of the diagnosis but I still didn't want a biopsy. My intuition was to try a treatment called Apheresis that I learned of from a colleague and friend, Rigdon Lentz, an oncologist. This treatment involves dialysis of a protein that almost all cancers make to shield them from the immune system, TNF-alpha Receptor. This molecule, also made by a human fetus to avoid rejection, blocks the normal activity of the tumor-destroying cytokine known as Tumor Necrosis Factor alpha (TNF) and thus ensures its survival. I knew his treatment was very safe and would allow my body to destroy any needle track spread of my cancer as well as other concerns I might harbor. Dr. Lentz agreed to treat me only if I had proof of cancer.

Even I though the Apheresis treatments were my best bet, I still wanted to avoid a biopsy. I saw a urologist who did a rectal exam and felt a mass on the right side of my prostate. I remembered a medical lecture by a urologist who used

HIFU (High Frequency Ultrasound) to treat prostate cancer. He said a biopsy wasn't necessary because his treatment would eradicate any present cancer and would not lead to urinary dribbling or impotence. I traveled to his Florida office and had another digital rectal exam, a prostate ultrasound and an MRI with Gadolinium enhancement. The tests revealed multiple suspicious masses, benign prostate hypertrophy and many calcium stones in my prostate. He advised me to undergo HIFU, for which would be done outside the U.S., and which would involve a TUR (trans urethral resection of my prostate gland) and necessitate a suprapubic cystostomy and catheter because he would destroy my urethra (he said it would grow back and the catheter would be removed in 10 days.) I was shocked and confused, as I thought I was going to undergo a very benign, safe procedure with guaranteed normal urinary and sexual function, and no cancer recurrence. I returned home.

I scheduled a biopsy with my urologist. Of the 12 cores taken, three were positive for malignancy with Gleason scores of 3+3, 3+3 and 3+4, and one core "suspicious for malignancy". I called Dr. Lentz and he said he would treat me but recommended some type of local treatment first. He listed radiation therapy, radiation seed implants, and then said he knew of another alternative—Transurethral Hyperthermia. He referred me to Ralf Kleef, M.D. in Vienna, Austria. Dr. Kleef kindly explained everything over the phone and I agreed to come over. The treatment consisted of the insertion of a Foley-type catheter with a heating element positioned so it rested in the prostatic portion of the urethra. The device is turned on and the treatment is raised to 50 degrees centigrade (122 degrees F). My treatment lasted 3 hours and was repeated two days later. The next day I was able to urinate like I could when I was 25 years old! I couldn't believe the strength of my steam.

Because I wanted to clean up any cancer cells that may have spread outside the prostate gland, I went to Dr. Lentz in Bavaria, Germany the next Monday after the treatment. He did a complete physical and the rectal exam was entirely normal—the tumor that had been palpated by the urologist was no longer felt!

I underwent five Apheresis treatments with a plan to go back after my parathyroid surgery. My PSA on 9/28/11 was 2.8. I underwent parathyroidectomy on November 3, 2011 and began feeling better almost immediately. My calcium dropped from 12.0 to 9.5 over four days. My PSA ranged from 3.3 to 5.5 over the next two months. I now was anxious to continue treatments for the prostate cancer, so I returned to Germany for eight more Apheresis treatments.

After returning home, I continued high dose vitamin C intravenous infusions and underwent 30 intravenous EDTA chelation treatment in the first four months of 2012 in order to flush out all of the calcium that had accumulated in my tissues overs the years due to Hyperparathyroidism.

After returning from Germany, I measured my PSA every month or so. It continued to vary from 3.3 to 6.5. Since the PCA-3 is more specific for cancer, I repeated it in February 2012. It was still elevated at 112. I saw my urologist that same month and he was amazed that he couldn't feel the mass he had palpated in 2011. In fact, he said, "Since you are already working outside of the box, I'm not recommending surgery." While that was good news, I decided to go back to Vienna and get some more hyperthermia because the PCA-3 was still elevated. To see if there was any improvement in the cancer areas of my gland, I had a repeat MRI just before the hyperthermia treatments. It revealed a reduction in the suspicious areas but one lesion remained visible. I went to Dr. Kleef's office and had two more hyperthermia treatments in June 2012.

While I was there, Dr. Kleef introduced me to Frank Gansauge, MD, PhD, a surgeon and immunologist. He offered dendritic cell vaccine therapy: it would use my own separated white blood cells that would then be grown in my own serum, where presumably any cancer antigens would be present. This "programs" the cells to identify such antigens, and when injected back in my body, they would kill any circulating cells so "tagged." I had the injection two weeks later.

I continued various nutritional and herbal therapies and followed my PSA as a general guide to judge if I had eradicated all of the cancer. The numbers varied between 5.8 and 8.4 but I knew that the treatments I had undergone might result in a temporary rise in the PSA. Still, I thought the PSA should eventually go below the 2008 level of 3.8, and became concerned when it didn't.

A colleague and a patient of mine both asked me if had seen Dr. Robert Bard, a radiologist in New York, who did sophisticated ultrasound exams that can not only reveal the presence of cancer, but also how malignant it might be based on the amount of blood flowing into it. I went to New York for his exam. It revealed two remaining areas with higher than normal vascularity. One was 14mm in diameter and of very high vascularity. Because of this, Dr. Bard thought I should consider MRI-guided laser destruction of the tumor by Dr. Daniel Sperling. I decided to see Dr. Sperling, whose MRI revealed only one tumor (the one seen on ultrasound by Dr. Bard). He was able to totally destroy the tumor with the MRI-guided laser treatment. After reviewing all three MRIs, Dr. Sperling said that the treatments

I had previously undergone had worked to eliminate all tumors except the one he then destroyed. He said I still had a lot of stones in my prostate, which could be the source of the ongoing elevated PSA. It of course went up to 17 after the laser procedure, and then went down to 6.1 one month later. He told me it may continue to be high for six months as a result of the treatment.

I am very glad I made the choice to forgo radical surgery or radiation therapy. Even these mutilating and potentially dangerous interventions cannot guarantee that the cancer won't come back. Prostate cancer will strike almost all men if they live long enough. Men should view it as a disease that can be managed, like diabetes. There is now good evidence that a plant-based diet, exercise program, body weight reduction and nutritional supplements, especially antioxidants, can stop the progression of prostate cancer and even reverse it in some cases. I hope to live out my life with an intact genitourinary system and practice a lifestyle that will prevent me from dying of cancer as well as enjoying a healthy life into old age. I am very grateful for the fine group of physicians who treated me.

April 15, 2013 – Edwin Kasten, D.C.

Dear Dr. Bard,

I would like to express my sincere gratitude for your knowledge, guidance and expertise during my journey with prostate cancer. Shortly after losing my wife to lung cancer, at a very humbling time in my life, I was diagnosed with prostate cancer. I was 62 years old at the time of diagnosis. Naturally I began to explore my options, which included a biopsy to determine the extent of the disease and was told I had a Gleason score of 7. After speaking with several Urologists, my options seemed bleak. They offered removal of the prostate gland, by conventional or Robotic assisted surgery, Radiation and hormone therapy. I did not want conventional surgery or therapies due to the physical and sexual side effects, which I was not prepared to live with.

As a Chiropractor, I have always believed in the body's ability to heal itself, if given the tools to do so. Vitamins and other supplements have always been a part of my daily routine. After being diagnosed, I increased my regimen of supplements hoping to prevent the disease from spreading. All the while, I continued searching for a more integrative, holistic approach. While searching on Dr. Joseph Mercola's website (mercola.com) I came upon his article that recommended Dr. Robert Bard. He went on to describe the state of the art ultrasound machine that Dr. Bard used to assist him in properly diagnosing the extent and measurement of the tumor(s). This type of testing can be done as often as necessary without the invasive use of needles, as in a biopsy. My secretary immediately made an appointment for me to have a consultation with Dr. Bard. It was my good fortune to find such a knowledgeable source for treatment and protocols in the area of prostate cancer. At the first visit, I was able to begin Dr. Bard's vitamin/supplement protocol and active surveillance. With his watchful eyes upon me, I was able to treat my cancer for over six years, until a better method of treatment was developed.

In December of 2012, at the age of 69, upon Dr. Bard's recommendation, I had Laser Ablation of the prostate gland. The procedure was done on a Friday and I returned to work on Monday with no side effects and no problems.

On Friday April 13, 2013 I had my five-month check up with Dr. Bard and I am elated to say I am cancer free. I wish to express my heartfelt gratitude to Dr. Bard for his tireless work in the area of cancer treatment along with his guidance and help during this trying time.

Sincerely,

Edwin Kasten, D.C.

Diplomate-American Board of Disability Analysts

March 2012 – Dr. Myron T.

Thank you for introducing me to Dr. Sperling. His laser treatment of my patients has been remarkable in its simplicity and efficacy. I will continue to refer my patients from British Columbia, Canada, to you both in the future.

Best regards,

Dr. Myron T.

August 4, 2005 – Ira G.

Dear Dr. Bard:

On June 29, 2005 I went to see you. Thanks to your expertise and very special equipment which provides 3-D imaging, you found that I had a virulent type of prostate cancer. You gave me a packet of materials on HIFU treatment—high intensity focused ultrasound. The treatment's 90 degree Celsius temperature destroys the cancer cells in seconds without side effects. Clearly, this is a major breakthrough in prostate cancer treatment.

Shortly thereafter I saw my urologist who scoffed at your findings of virulence. He said emphatically that this could not be determined. Also that 97 percent of prostate cancers are benign. Especially, since I am 94, he advised me to sit tight. If the situation worsened badly, radiation could be used.

Radiation did not seem to me much of an option. It involves a considerable blood loss, and I have anemia and heart problems.

My Urologist's advice plainly was based on probability—that 97 percent of prostate cancers are benign. But probability doesn't apply to a single event, such as one case. His advice involved a gamble, one contrary to your findings that I was among the 3 percent: Speed in treatment was essential. HIFU is available only before the cancer has metastasized.

Time was not on my side. On July 31 I underwent treatment in Cancun, Mexico at an American Hospital. My doctor George M. Suarez—a Miami, FL based American urologist/surgeon painlessly blitzed the cancer with high intensity focused ultrasound. Three hours later in the recovery room he informed me that cancer had not metastasized and that I was cancer free.

Widely practiced for years in Europe, Asia, Canada and elsewhere, in the US HIFU—at long last, is in FDA's third stage trials. Hopefully, this important technological advance will soon be available here.

Ira G.

NOTE: Mr. G. passed away 1 day before 100th birthday from a stroke. Dr. Bard

August 15, 2006 – Alan

Good morning Dr. Bard,

Since July 17, 2006, I have been taking ProMultiCell 2 capsules 3x per day as you recommended for my prostate cancer. I have type 2 diabetes; I take 1000 mg. of Metformin twice daily, along with 5 mg. of Glipizide once daily. My blood sugar level has been hovering around 130-160, which is higher than I would like. Since I've been taking your ProMultiCell formula, I've noticed a substantial decrease in my blood sugar level. The low was 63 with a high of 125. This morning after fasting it was 103. I've had readings in the morning of 73 and the afternoon and evening of 125-135. Those are great readings. I have not had such low readings for about three years. Last week in the afternoon I checked my blood sugar level it was 165. I took two ProMultiCell capsules and waited for one hour. I took another reading, it was down to 114.

Have you had an experience like this with any other diabetic patients? This is remarkable; I want to thank you for recommending ProMultiCell.

I had HIFU on July 23, 2006; it was performed in Toronto by Dr. George Suarez. It went very well, painless and so far no visible side effects. I have an appointment scheduled with you in January 2007; I am looking forward to seeing you then.

Thank you very much for all your help. Dr. Suarez was right when he said to me that you are a doctor ahead of your time.

Yours truly,

Alan

TEXT OF HRICAK PROSTATE PRESENTATION; ORNISH ABSTRACT

MRI, MR Spectroscopy and Computed Tomography of Prostate Cancer: An Update at the 2005 NY Roentgen Society Meeting

Hedvig Hricak, MD, PhD

Chairman, Department of Radiology,

Carroll and Milton Petrie Chair

Memorial Sloan-Kettering Cancer Center

Professor of Radiology,

Weill Medical College of Cornell University

Prostate cancer is the most common cancer and the second leading cause of cancer death in American men. Given its biological heterogeneity, the high prevalence of indolent disease, and the desire for patient-specific treatment design, non-invasive evaluation of tumor prognostic variables, including tumor location, volume, aggressiveness, and extent, continues to be of great clinical interest. Magnetic resonance imaging (MRI) and spectroscopic imaging (MRSI) have demonstrated potential in localizing prostate cancer lesions and assessing tumor aggressiveness and extent. CT has been found helpful in the evaluation of metastatic prostate cancer in radiotherapy planning and treatment follow-up. These modalities can therefore play an important role in risk-adjusted, patient-specific treatment selection, planning and follow-up.

Role of MRI/MRSI in Pretreatment Assessment of Prostate Cancer

Although biopsy is considered the preferred method for prostate cancer detection and characterization, data suggest that even with a threshold PSA value of 4.1 ng per milliliter, biopsy will miss 82% of cancers in men less than 60 years old and 65% of cancers in men over 60. In fact, when biopsy results were compared with radical prostatectomy for sextant tumor localization, the positive predictive value of biopsy was 83.3%, and the negative predictive value was 36.4%. MRI/MRSI is not recommended as a first approach to diagnose prostate cancer but may be useful for directing targeted biopsy, especially for patients with PSA levels indicative of cancer but with negative previous biopsy results; this situation occurs most often with lesions in the anterior peripheral or transition zones (i.e., regions not palpable by digital rectal examination (DRE) and often not routinely sampled during biopsy). The combined use of MRI and MRSI has shown excellent sensitivity and specificity for detecting cancer in the peripheral zone. In a recent study comparing DRE, transrectal ultrasound (TRUS)-guided biopsy and endorectal MRI in the detection and localization of prostate cancer, MRI performed significantly better than DRE in detecting cancer in the apex, mid-gland, and base, and significantly better than TRUS-guided biopsy in the mid gland and base. Unlike either DRE or TRUS-guided biopsy, MRI was also capable of detecting tumor in the transition zone. The use of MRI/MRSI may reduce the rate of false-negative biopsies and hence decrease the need for more extensive biopsy protocols and multiple repeat biopsy procedures.

One of the most challenging characteristics of prostate cancer is its variability in biological aggressiveness. Gleason grade is a good predictor of prostate cancer aggressiveness. However, biopsy prediction of final pathological grade is not reliable. As compared with the histology results from radical prostatectomy, biopsy determined the correct Gleason grade at best in only 58% of cases. MR spectroscopy has the potential to provide a noninvasive means of improving the assessment of prostate cancer aggressiveness. It has been shown that the ratio of choline+creatine to citrate in a prostate cancer lesion correlates with the Gleason grade, with the elevation of choline and reduction of citrate indicating increased tumor aggressiveness.

MRI/MRSI has also been shown to aid in determining the local extent of prostate cancer. A study by Wang et al. has shown that MRI contributes significant incremental value to clinical variables in the prediction of extracapsular extension. On MRI, the criteria for extracapsular extension include a contour deformity with a step-off or angulated margin; an irregular bulge or edge retraction; a breach of the capsule with evidence of direct tumor extension; obliteration of the recto-prostatic angle; and asymmetry of the neurovascular bundles. While transaxial planes of section are essential in the evaluation of extracapsular invasion, the combination of transaxial and coronal plane images facilitates the diagnosis of extracapsular extension. The addition of volumetric data from MRSI to the anatomic display of MRI significantly improves the evaluation of extracapsular cancer extension and decreases interobserver variability.

MRI is also useful for demonstrating seminal vesicle invasion. The criteria for seminal vesicle invasion on MRI include contiguous low signal-intensity tumor extension from the base of the gland into the seminal vesicles; tumor extension along the ejaculatory duct (non-visualization of the ejaculatory duct); asymmetric decrease in the signal intensity of the seminal vesicles; and decreased conspicuity of the seminal vesicle wall on T2-weighted images. Combined axial, coronal and sagittal planes of section facilitate evaluation of seminal vesical and bladder neck invasion.

Over the past four years, studies on the use MRI in the evaluation of prostate cancer have obtained more promising results than did initial studies. The diagnostic performance for experienced readers has improved, with reported accuracy reaching between 75% and 93%. The recently reported sensitivities of MRI for detection of extracapsular extension and seminal vesicle invasion and the high specificity of MRI in excluding extracapsular tumors far exceed the values reported for both TRUS and CT. However, it has been shown that the incremental value of MRI in predicting extracapsular extension is significant only when interpretation is performed by a radiologist with substantial experience in MRI and thorough clinical knowledge of the disease. This suggests that the recent improvement in the performance of MRI is likely due to increased reader experience in addition to the maturation of MRI technology (e.g. faster imaging sequences, more powerful gradient coils, and post-processing image correction) and better understanding of morphologic criteria used to diagnose extracapsular extension or seminal vesicle invasion.

Computed Tomography

The main role of CT in prostate cancer management is in the assessment of metastatic disease in the lymph nodes, visceral organs and bones. Due to the lack of soft-tissue contrast, CT has limited value in initial tumor staging, unless advanced disease is suspected. However, it is useful in radiotherapy treatment planning in patients with locally advanced prostate cancer and also in treatment follow-up. The majority of patients with newly diagnosed prostate cancer are at low risk for metastases, hence the diagnostic yield of CT is relatively low in these patients. CT is not recommended for patients with a PSA < 20 ng/ml, a Gleason score < 7, or a clinical stage < T3 as the likelihood of lymph node metastasis and systemic disease is very low. At present, according to the American Urology Association guidelines, there is no indication for CT in a patient with a PSA level < 25 ng/ml.

CT Imaging Findings in Local Tumor Staging

Although there is no recent literature on the CT appearance of organ-confined prostate cancer, in our personal experience with multi-slice CT, prostate cancer appears as an area of low attenuation compared to the surrounding normal prostate tissue. CT can be useful as a baseline examination prior to radiation or medical therapy in clinically high-risk patients with grossly advanced local disease demonstrated by established extracapsular disease, gross seminal vesicle invasion, or invasion of surrounding structures including bladder, rectum, levator ani muscles, or pelvic floor. Such patients will also be at risk for lymph node metastases, which may be assessed concurrently.

Detection of Metastatic Disease on CT

Currently, the diagnosis of nodal metastases on CT is made based on nodal size. However, the correlation between nodal enlargement and metastatic involvement is poor. Using a short axis diameter of 1.0 cm as a cut off has resulted in sensitivity values between 25% and 85% and specificity between 66% and 100%. Oyen et al reported a significant improvement in both sensitivity and specificity (78% and 100% respectively) with lowering of the size threshold to 0.7 cm and performance of fine needle aspiration (FNA) of the suspicious nodes. However, neither decreased size criteria, nor the use of FNA has been widely accepted. Neither CT nor MRI can be used to rule out lymph node metastases, especially in normal-sized lymph nodes. However, recently, high-resolution MRI with lymphotropic superparamagnetic nanoparticles has demonstrated promising results in diagnosis of metastasis within normal-sized lymph nodes.

Knowledge of the anatomical nodal spread is essential for proper image interpretation. The regional nodes for prostate cancer that are designated as N1 in the TNM classification are pelvic nodes, including obturator, iliac (internal and external), and sacral (lateral, presacral, promontory) nodes. Metastatic lymph nodes (M1) are common iliac, paraaortic, mesenteric and mediastinal nodes. Prior to any form of therapy, nodal disease usually progresses in step-wise fashion, such that retroperitoneal, mesenteric or mediastinal nodal disease is very unusual in the absence of pelvic lymphadenopathy and more likely to be due to coexistent malignancy (e.g., lymphoma). However, in patients with disease recurrence following radical prostatectomy the usual pattern of vertical node spread is not maintained in almost 75% of the patients. The majority of these patients would have had previous lymph node dissection at the time of radical prostatectomy and thus only retroperitoneal lymphadenopathy would be detected at CT.

CT is also valuable in the evaluation of visceral and bone metastasis. Bone metastases from prostate cancer are usually sclerotic due to osteoblastic reaction, but a mixed lytic-sclerotic pattern can occasionally be observed. However, bone scintigraphy and MRI are superior to CT in since metastasis after chemo/radiation treatment can appear larger, thus leading to incorrect estimation of disease progression.

ABSTRACT of Dean Ornish, MD 2005 paper in the *Journal of Urology*

Title: Intensive Lifestyle Changes May Affect the Progression of Prostate Cancer
    Conclusions:

"Patients...maintain comprehensive lifestyle changes...resulting in significant decreases in serum PSA"

"...substantially decreased growth of LNCaP prostate cancer cells was seen when such cells were incubated in the presence of serum from those who made lifestyle changes. These findings suggest that intensive changes in diet and lifestyle may beneficially affect the progression of early prostate cancer."

APPENDIX D

RESOURCES

INTERNET NUTRITIONAL RESOURCES

Arbor Clinical Nutrition Updates
http://www.nutritionupdates.org/

Center for Responsible Nutrition
http://www.crnusa.org/

American Holistic Medical Association
www.holisticmedicine.org

Consumer Lab:
http://consumerlab.com

FDA Center for Food Safety & Applied Nutrition
http://www.cfsan.fda.gov/

Food and Nutrition Information Center
http://www.nal.usda.gov/fnic

NIH National Center for Complementary and Alternative Medicine:
http://nccam.nih.gov

NIH Office of Dietary Supplements
http://dietary-suplements.info.nih.gov

Breaking news on supplements and nutrition
http://www.nutraingredients-usa.com/

SupplementWatch
http://www.supplementwatch.com/

The American Herbal Pharmacopoeia
http://www.herbal-ahp.org/

Harvard Women's Healthwatch
http://www.health.harvard.edu/newsletters/Harvard_Womens_Health_Watch.htm

Mayo Clinic Newsletter
www.mayoclinic.com

PUBLICATIONS
Journals and Magazines
Alternative and Complementary Therapies info@liebertpub.com
Mary Ann Liebert, Inc. Publishers www.liebertpub.com
2 Madison Ave,
Larchmont, NY 10538
(914) 834-3100

Journal of Medicinal Foods http://www.liebertonline.com/jmf
Alternative Therapies in Health and Medicine http://www.alternative-therapies.com
InnoVision Communications, LLC
2995 Wilderness Place, Suite 205
Boulder, CO 80301
(303) 440-7402

EXPLORE: The Journal of Science and Healing http://www.explorejournal.com/
Elsevier Inc.
360 Park Avenue South
New York, NY 10010
(800) 654-2452

HerbalGram www.herbalgram.org
American Botanical Council
PO BOX 2016600
Austin, TX 78720
(512) 926-4900

Newsletters and Other Periodicals
Center for Medical Consumers www.medicalconsumers.org
239 Thompson St. medconsumers@earthlink.net
New York, NY 10012

The Collaborative on Health and the Environment www.healthandenvironment.
org
c/o Commonweal
PO Box 316, Bolinas, CA 94924

Environmental Nutrition http://www.environmentalnutrition.com/
P.O. Box 420234
Palm Coast, FL 32142-0234
800-829-5384

OTHER RESOURCES
American Botanical Council www.herbalgram.org
PO Box 201660
Austin, TX 78720-1660
(512) 331-886 (800)-373-7105

ARTICLES FOR YOUR INTEREST

You Can Spark Your Creativity

Thomas Edison remains America's greatest innovator. While other inventors spend their lives working on a single breakthrough—or simply stumble upon an invention—Edison was a master of innovative thinking. He held more than 1,000 patents during his life, more than any other person in the nation's history.

There may be only one Edison, but we all can develop our innovation skills. By learning these bright lessons from him, we can boost our creativity and solve professional and personal problems.

Use what you learn. Many of Edison's breakthroughs were the result of taking an idea from one field and applying it to something entirely different. Using carbon to boost telephone transmitter volume came from his earlier attempt to study resistance in electrical cables. That cable experiment was unsuccessful— carbon's resistance changed too easily to meet his needs—but while working on phone transmitters, it occurred to Edison that carbon was just what was needed to replicate sound waves. His resulting innovation was a crucial part of every phone until the digital age.

Look at the big picture. Edison didn't just invent the electric light. His company also built the electricity-generating infrastructure to run the lights, complete with power stations and transmission wires. It came as no surprise to Edison that power generation became a more profitable industry than bulb manufacturing—people buy bulbs only now and then, but they pay to run them every day. Building an integrated power system also gave Edison an advantage over competitors, who had to build lights that would work on his system.

Explore ideas. Some of Edison's discoveries came from experiments that were meant simply to increase his knowledge. He made a crucial breakthrough on his electric light while experimenting with heating metals. Edison believed that the key to an electric light lay in finding the right filament—but during his experiments with metal, he was struck by the effect of impurities in the metal. It occurred to him that impurities in the air around the filament could be significant. He decided to put his filament in a vacuum. Sealed-air light bulbs remain in use to this day.

Find a kernel of success in failure. Edison used to say that he never had a failed experiment. Even when experiments went wrong, they still boosted his knowledge.

Example: Edison poured a huge amount of time and money into an ore-milling company, only to see the venture fail when ore discoveries in the Midwest reduced prices. The ore operation has been widely regarded as Edison's greatest folly. Before the company failed, though, Edison noted that the sand that was a by-product of ore milling could be sold to cement makers. Seeing an opportunity, Edison soon entered the cement industry, patenting substantial improvements in both rock-crushing and kiln technologies. He received royalties on every barrel of cement produced from kilns of his design. His company even supplied the cement for the original Yankee Stadium. None of this would have happened if Edison simply had written off ore milling as a failure.

Keep improving. Edison often spent years refining his ideas. Continued innovation enabled him to stay ahead of his competitors by lowering manufacturing costs and improving quality.

Example: Edison filed more patents related to electric lights in 1882 than in any other year—even though he had already perfected the practical incandescent lamp three years earlier.

One reason why Edison was able to refine his ideas was that he didn't sell the rights to his inventions—his company manufactured and sold his products. Edison used feedback from customers, salespeople and engineers to perfect his designs.

Effect of nutritional supplement challenge in patients with isolated high-grade prostatic intraepithelial neoplasia

(<u>Urology.</u> 2007 Jun;69(6):1102-6.)

Joniau S, Goeman L, Roskams T, Lerut E, Oyen R, Van Poppel H. (Department of Urology, University Hospitals Katholieke Universiteit Leuven, Leuven, Belgium)

OBJECTIVES: To investigate, through a prospective follow-up study, the effects of a dietary supplementation challenge in men with isolated high-grade prostatic intraepithelial neoplasia (HGPIN)

METHODS: The effects of a 6-month supplementation challenge with selenium, vitamin E, and soy isoflavonoids in men diagnosed with isolated HGPIN on biopsy were evaluated. A total of 100 patients entered the study. Of the 100 men, 29 were excluded because they refused additional biopsies or were noncompliant with the protocol, 71 underwent repeat biopsies at 3 months, and 58 underwent a third set at 6 months. The prostate-specific antigen (PSA) level was recorded at inclusion and before each set of biopsies. The study endpoint was defined as the diagnosis of PCa at 3 months or the histopathologic status at 6 months.

RESULTS: At the study endpoint, PCa had been found in 24 men (33.8%), HGPIN in 34 (47.9%), and no HGPIN or carcinoma in 13 (18.3%). The PCa risk throughout the study period was 25.0% in the group with a stable or decreasing PSA level (n = 48, 67.6%) and 52.2% in the group with an increasing PSA level (n = 23, 32.4%). This difference was statistically significant (P = 0.0458). Isolated HGPIN remaining at the first repeat biopsy and the percentage of initial cores with HGPIN were significant predictors of PCa at additional biopsies.

CONCLUSIONS: The results of our study have shown that a decrease in the PSA level while taking a selenium, vitamin E, and soy isoflavonoids supplement predicts for a significantly lower risk of PCa in future biopsies. The percentage of initial biopsy cores with HGPIN and isolated HGPIN remaining at the first repeat biopsy are significant predictors of PCa in future biopsies.

MID: 17572195 [PubMed–indexed for MEDLINE]

Dutasteride Results Reignite Debate
About Prevention of Prostate Cancer

March 31, 2010 (Reported online at <u>http://www.medscape.com/viewarticle/719549</u>)

New results showing that dutasteride (*Avodart*, GlaxoSmithKline) reduces the risk for prostate cancer have propelled the subject of chemoprevention for prostate cancer into the spotlight once again.

But the latest results do not convince an expert who has spoken out against this approach in the past; he does so again in an editorial accompanying the study in the March 31 issue of the *New England Journal of Medicine*.

The study, known as Reduction by Dutasteride of Prostate Cancer Events (REDUCE), was conducted in men considered to be at a high risk for prostate cancer because of their age (50 to 75 years of age), an elevated level of prostate-specific antigen (PSA), or because they had already had a prostate biopsy because of suspicion of prostate cancer.

Over the course of 4 years, significantly fewer prostate cancers were detected in men taking dutasteride than in those taking placebo, representing a relative risk reduction of 22.8% ($P < .001$).

The researchers, headed by Gerald Andriole, MD, chief of urologic surgery at Washington University School of Medicine in St. Louis, Missouri, conclude that dutasteride "may be considered as a treatment option for men who are at high risk of prostate cancer."

The data from this trial, which was sponsored by the manufacturer of dutasteride, have been submitted for approval for the indication of prostate cancer risk reduction, Dr. Andriole told *Medscape Oncology*. Currently, dutasteride is marketed for use in benign prostatic hyperplasia.

Nothing New?

Editorialist Patrick Walsh, MD, from the James Buchanan Brady Urological Institute at Johns Hopkins Medical Institutions in Baltimore, Maryland, told *Medscape Oncology* that the new data on dutasteride are similar to what has been seen with finasteride (*Proscar*, Merck & Co), and he believes that neither drug should be prescribed for the chemoprevention of prostate cancer.

"Dutasteride and finasteride do not prevent prostate cancer, but merely temporarily shrink tumors that have a low potential for being lethal," Dr. Walsh writes in his editorial. "Furthermore, the use of these drugs for prevention may be somewhat risky," he warned. These drugs suppress PSA levels, Dr. Walsh told *Medscape Oncology*. This is "worrisome," he explained, because a decrease in PSA might convince men that the drug is preventing prostate cancer and lull them into a false sense of security that could delay a diagnosis "until they have disease that is difficult to cure," he said.

"Major Distinction" Between Findings

Dr. Andriole agreed that the broad results for the 2 drugs are similar â€" dutasteride was shown to reduce the risk for prostate cancer by 23%, which is close to the 25% reduction seen with finasteride.

But there is a "major distinction" between the 2 drugs in the findings of high-grade tumors, he told *Medscape Oncology*. This has been a major concern with the finasteride data. The 7-year Prostate Cancer Prevention Trial found a reduction in low-grade tumors, but at the same time found an increase in high-grade tumors in the drug group over the placebo group. However, later analyses suggested that the effect of finasteride that reduced the size of the prostate made these high-grade tumors easier to find, rather than increasing their incidence.

In the just-published REDUCE trial, Dr. Andriole said there was "no increase in high-grade tumors in the raw data."

Although the numbers show a significant increase in high-grade tumors in the dutasteride group, compared with the placebo group (12 vs 1; $P\hat{A}$ = .003), Dr. Andriole asserted that this imbalance can be explained by the men in the placebo group being excluded from the trial if their first biopsy found a tumor. If those men had remained in the study and been biopsied again a few years later, some of their tumors "likely would have been upgraded," he explained, and this would have resulted in the number of high-grade tumors in the 2 groups being comparable. "This so-called tumor upgrading has been observed in other studies," he said, adding that this point is elaborated upon in the discussion section of their paper.

Dr. Andriole also noted that if the mathematical modeling that was applied to the finasteride data was applied to the dutasteride data, it would actually show a statistically significant 38% reduction in the risk for high-grade tumors. This is not detailed in their paper, but is explained in a supplementary appendix, he said.

Recommended for Men at High Risk

Dr. Andriole told *Medscape Oncology* that he recommends prescribing dutasteride to men who are at high risk for prostate cancer (because of elevated levels of PSA, such as in this trial, or because of a family history of the disease). "This drug can reduce the man's chance of being overdiagnosed and overtreated for prostate cancer," he added.

In addition, he believes that the benefits of reducing the risk for prostate cancer and the improvement seen in outcomes related to benign prostatic hyperplasia outweigh the risk for adverse effects, which include sexual dysfunction and, in this trial, heart failure.

The sexual adverse effects, which include erectile dysfunction (reported in 9% of men taking dutasteride and in 5.7% of men taking placebo; $P\hat{A} < .001$), are reversible, Dr. Andriole said, and if they do appear, the drug can be discontinued, he added. Heart failure (reported in 0.7% of men taking dutasteride and in 0.4% of men taking placebo; $P\hat{A} = .03$) has not been reported as an adverse effect with these drugs, he noted. He suspects that the cases seen in this trial are related to the concomitant use of alpha blockers, although he admitted that this is "speculation."

Use Recommended by ASCO and AUA

The American Society of Clinical Oncology (ASCO) and the American Urological Association (AUA) jointly recommended the use of both dutasteride and finasteride in asymptomatic men to reduce the risk for prostate cancer in new guidelines issued in February 2009.

However, to date there has been little use of these drugs for this indication, several experts have told *Medscape Oncology* in previous interviews. This is an off-label use at present; both drugs are marketed for benign prostatic hypertrophy (finasteride is also marketed for male pattern baldness).

Dr. Andriole agreed that there has been little use of finasteride for reducing the risk for prostate cancer, and believes that this stems from concern over the high-grade tumor findings. He believes that the new data on dutasteride will "lay that anxiety to rest," and that these latest data will lead to an increase in the use of dutasteride for this indication.

Expert Discourages Use for Prevention

Dr. Walsh is firmly opposed to the use of these drugs for prostate cancer risk reduction. He has spoken out against finasteride in comments made in response to an article about the drug preventing cancer that made the front page of the *New York Times* (June 15, 2008). "I am very concerned about encouraging patients and general physicians to use this drug," he wrote in the Winter 2009 issue of *Prostate Cancer Discovery.* He notes finasteride does not prevent prostate cancer, "it just prevents men from knowing they have it!"

"First, it has no primary effect in reducing the number of men who will have a positive biopsy," he writes. "Second, men will believe that it prevents cancer, will be pleased that their PSA levels fall, and will not understand the potential danger of undiagnosed high-grade disease."

Dr. Walsh told *Medscape Oncology* that the comments he made about finasteride at that time apply equally to dutasteride.

"[REDUCE] showed that there was a 23% reduction in low-grade tumors that the patients would never have known they had," he said. "Does this sound like an indication to take a pill with sexual side effects that costs $4 a day?"

In his editorial, Dr. Walsh reviews previous studies on finasteride and the latest study on dutasteride. He points out that neither drug "significantly reduced the risk of prostate cancer among men who were followed closely and who underwent a biopsy because of an elevated PSA level (corrected for the effect of the drug) or an abnormal digital rectal examination." He adds that, "unfortunately, this is the setting that would be used for prevention."

But this approach "will continue to be pushed because of financial interests," he told *Medscape Oncology*. The clinical trials have been huge and the companies involved "must have spent a ton of money on it," he noted.

A discussion of these latest results and the implications for clinical practice has just been published on a Medscape blog entitled *Controversies in Urology*.

The REDUCE trial was supported by GlaxoSmithKline, manufacturer of dutasteride, and 4 of the coauthors are employees of the company. Dr. Andriole reports receiving consulting or advisory fees from GlaxoSmithKline and 8 other pharmaceutical companies; several coauthors report receiving consulting, advisory, or lecture fees from GlaxoSmithKline. Details are in the paper. Dr. Walsh has disclosed no relevant financial relationships.

N Engl J Med. 2010; 363; 1192-1202, 1237-1238.

Since the last publication of this text, two (2) US patents have been issued regarding the anti-oxidant treatment of prostate cancer. This summarizes the pertinent features of these patented formulations.

Advances in Cancer Imaging and Treatment

NOTE: In addition to the content of this article, it is important to know that detection and monitoring by means of Doppler ultrasound may help men avoid biopsies if DRE is negative and PSA is less than 10. R. Bard

Diagnosing, Treating and Reversing Prostate and other Cancers with Non-Invasive Monitoring and Nutritional Intervention: Minimally Invasive Biopsy and Treatment Options

By Robert Bard MD

Director, Biofoundation for Angiogenesis; Assoc.

Professor Radiology, NY Medical College

Introduction

A primary goal in prostate and other cancers is to identify aggressive cancers that can kill, as opposed to cancers that do not threaten life, and may not even show any symptoms. The current, widely-used diagnostic techniques make this identification extremely elusive. The technology to achieve this diagnostic distinction should be noninvasive, and provide measures that can be easily and accurately compared to previous exams, making it easy to track changes. At the same time, it should provide a systematic approach to monitoring the patient's response to therapeutic intervention. In this way the diagnosis, monitoring and treatment can be tailored to each individual's circumstances and responsiveness.

With recent advances in the technology of Doppler ultrasound and MRI, these goals can and are being achieved. Until recently this diagnostic technology has required extensive experience and training in interpreting the images. Now, advances in the computerization of the imaging, blood flow, and tumor measures of exact size and density, provide for an accurate and repeatable diagnosis, and a means to follow the individual's unique pattern of cancer development, progress, and response to treatment. Recent technological advances also make these procedures available to much broader clinical application, without requiring years of very unique training and experience, and these advances are applicable beyond prostate cancer (PCa), the example used here.

In this paper, the noninvasive diagnostic tracking of a patient's progress is presented, along with a naturopathic nutritional approach, the Beta-Sitosterol/Antioxidant Matrix (B-Sit/AOX), which provides vital support for cell function and membrane integrity. The B-Sit/AOX Matrix properly restores essential nutrition that has been systematically removed from our food supply.

It systemically supports the body, and is especially targeted to naturally restore cell membrane elasticity and permeability, apoptosis, reduce cell proliferation, and reestablish a healthy intracellular environment that naturally protects against metastases. This directly nourishes the body's natural cancer prevention mechanisms, and is appropriate for healthy individuals, for individuals during cancer episodes, and for post-episode maintenance. Following men with PCa using Doppler imaging has shown that an appropriate B-Sit/AOX formulation is effective and successful for a wide range of men with diagnosed prostate cancer who elect proactive watchful waiting. The evaluation of nearly 10 years of patient records for men opting for proactive watchful waiting (Gleason scores ranging from 5 to 9) using the B-Sit/AOX Matrix has demonstrated the success of this nutritional approach—with the result being approximately 90% of men showed significant reduction or full stabilization of vascular indices for non-aggressive cancers, and the same improvement was shown in nearly 70% of men with aggressive cancers, over a ten year period. Careful monitoring also provides the basis for deciding on other available treatment options, if necessary.

The success of coupling noninvasive monitoring with key nutrition provides a robust basis for tailoring intervention to an individual. This system provides a reliable evaluation of each person on a case-by-case criterion. Thus we are able to evaluate the individual's ability to respond to nutritional and life-style intervention, and the potential need for more invasive medical intervention and treatment, while reducing unnecessary invasive treatments.

Background & Brief History:

In 1940, the classic textbook of pathology, Ewing's NEOPLASTIC DISEASES[1] noted prostate cancer is a rare disease, accounting for 2.7 % of tumors in the male population of that era. Half a century ago, pathologists found a high percentage of men without "clinical" prostate cancer to have malignant cells in the operative specimens of surgery for relief of benign prostatic obstruction. In addition, the rate of cancer being present in prostates examined during autopsy varies dramatically in different regions of the world, with the food supply being the single variable able to account for the differences. In the absence of demonstrable tumor invasion, perhaps cancer formation should be considered a non-threatening aspect of normal body aging, or at worst, a chronic disease that is governed by lifestyle and the available food supply.

This leads to a simple clinical question: Is there a way to determine whether a cancer is part of the natural aging process to be watched (inconsequential cancer) or whether the malignancy will have deadly consequences?

This question is being answered by a building body of knowledge that has recently been accelerated by technological advances in diagnostic imaging. In 1985, a prominent British physician, David Cosgrove, published a paper in the *American Journal of Radiology* demonstrating the presence of blood flows in breast cancers. The new generation of sonogram equipment had the capability to show pictures of blood vessels. The arteries and veins supplying a tumor could be clearly imaged. Moreover, the actual flowing blood in the cancer could be seen and velocity of flow of blood in the vessels accurately measured. At an international conference in Italy in 1997, Dr. Rodolfo Campani, an Italian radiologist specializing in studying the blood flows of cancers at the University of Pavia Medical Center, showed the criteria to differentiate malignant cancer vessels from benign tumor blood vessels. Benign vessels are few in number, smoothly outlined, follow straight courses and branch regularly. Malignant vessels are many in number, irregularly outlined, irregular in course and crooked in branching patterns. These findings have been confirmed by other investigators, and presented at the 2006 World Congress of Interventional Oncology. Today, malignant blood vessels may be accurately and non invasively detected by newer Doppler sonography techniques and advanced blood flow MRI protocols.

SONOGRAPHY:

Doppler Ultrasound has Wide Application for Improving Cancer Therapy

The physical principle of ultrasound, the piezoelectric effect where sound is created from electrical energy, was discovered by Pierre and Marie Curie ten years before the recognition of the X-Ray. Early medical uses included imaging disorders of the eye, heart and the developing fetus. As computers grew in sophistication, so did the applications of ultrasound, and now, it is often used as the first diagnostic test for many medical disorders. Doppler sonar created in 1972 gives pictures of flow movement in the human body in the same way it shows motion in the weather patterns (Doppler radar) that one sees on television weather reports. Doppler technology has been around for years.

Urologists in Japan, oncologists in England, surgeons in the Netherlands, chemotherapists in Belgium, ultrasonographers in Norway and radiologists in France, seeing the success of sonograms in diagnosing malignant tumors in the breast, turned their attention to the study of the prostate. They concluded that the vascular pattern shown by the Doppler technique held the key to the degree of malignancy. In 2002, German surgeons at the University of Ulm, the largest bone tumor center in Europe, showed bone cancers that were highly malignant had high blood flows. The current clinical use of Doppler equipment in Europe is keeping patients from unnecessarily losing their arms and legs to surgery. Historically, the standard treatment for bone cancer has been amputation of the entire limb, Current surgical intervention has become more conservative, often removing a limited portion of the bone so the tumor can be removed with a rim of normal bone without the need for an amputation. However, by distinguishing cancer aggressiveness, Doppler techniques have refined this even more, since bone tumors that demonstrate no vascularity or low blood flows are now watched or treated more conservatively.

Dr. Nathalie Lassau, an interventional radiologist at the Institute de Cancerologie Gustav Roussy, an internationally known cancer center in Paris, published similar findings on the deadly skin cancer, melanoma. Her article in the *American Journal of Radiology* in 2002[2] revealed lethal skin cancers to be highly vascular and skin cancers that could be watched were not vascular. Dr. Lassau is currently investigating medicines to reduce blood flows to cancers in hope of lessening their malignant consequences and has presented this work at numerous international meetings. Her finding that 3D Doppler sonography correlates best with the pathologic process was highlighted at the 2011, Eighth International Symposium on Melanoma. Now, newer MRI imaging protocols are currently being fine tuned based on the proven high accuracy of the Doppler sonography data.

Clinical Application of 3-D Doppler and MRI Diagnostic Technology

Imaging Aggressiveness: The blood flow patterns depicted by Doppler sonography provide a way to quantitatively measure and serially monitor the severity of malignancy, as well as the response to therapy throughout the treatment course. Blood flow analysis can show which cancers are aggressive, since these have many vessels and which are responding to treatment, or nutritional intervention, or both, since the number of tumor vessels decreases with successful therapies.[3]

Monitoring Intervals: Because it is a non-invasive procedure, the 3-D Doppler exam can be performed as often as necessary. Our experience has shown that cancers are more variable in their respond to intervention than generally believed. During early stages of diagnosis and intervention for PCa, a 3 month follow-up exam is warranted. Once the cancer shows signs of regressing, based primarily on measures of vascularity and density, a six to nine month follow-up schedule is more appropriate. MRIs should be repeated when…the tumor has not responded to treatment by six months. Routine ultrasound follow up should be on a 6 month basis and MRI yearly for 3 years.

Tumor Size Alone Can Be Misleading: The routine use of tumor size decrease has been shown to be less reliable than blood flow analysis, since the edema of cell death may cause dying cancers to enlarge. Although this concept was described in the early 1990's in Europe, it was first mentioned in the American literature in 1996 at the American Roentgen Ray Society Annual Meeting. Dr. E. Louvar from the Henry Ford Hospital combined radiology and pathology studies to determine that the power Doppler flows in malignancies was related to the vessels that fed aggressive tumors.

Highly Correlated to Gleason Scores: Significantly higher Gleason scores were seen in cancer biopsies of high Doppler flow areas compared to cancers with no Doppler flows. Dr. D. Downey at John Robarts Research Institute of the University Hospital in Ontario, Canada has looked at vascular imaging techniques and 3-dimensional imaging of blood vessels. Blood vessels can be rendered in 3-D with angiography (high intensity dye injected into arteries), CT scanning (medium intensity dye), MR angiography (low intensity dye), 3-D color Doppler imaging and 3-D power Doppler imaging. In this article published from the *American Journal of Radiology* in 1995, he noted that in prostate cancers power Doppler was better able to delineate the abnormal vessel architecture than color Doppler techniques. Indeed, computer analysis of malignant vessel density is now being used as a substitute for Gleason grading, which is solely based on randomly obtained histologic microscopic findings.

Clinical Advantage of Doppler Technologies: 3-D Doppler Ultrasound Overcomes Diagnostic Problems Caused by Treatments

Treatment Alters Standard Diagnostic Accuracy: A 2004 newsletter from the Prostate Cancer Research Institute reported that hormone therapy may change the way the pathologist interprets a cancer. Androgen deprivation therapy, (ADT) and similar medicines such as Proscar (finasteride), Avodart (dutasteride) and certain hair maintenance formulations, make it more difficult to grade the tumor with microscopic analysis. Dr. Pam Unger, a prostate cancer pathology specialist at Mount Sinai Hospital in New York, mentioned in a personal communication that radiation changes also caused difficulties in reading the microscopic slides. Furthermore, pathologists generally don't look for blood vessels, and thus, do not routinely evaluate the vascular pattern in the specimens they interpret.

Blood Flow, Measured by Doppler Sonogram, is Not Disrupted by Treatments: The diagnostic accuracy of 3-D Doppler, based on blood flow analysis, is not altered by the treatments noted above. Men who have been on ADT should have a Doppler sonogram study to confirm the absence of residual disease. If there are areas of abnormal blood vessels, biopsy may be considered. Many patients who have been treated for cancer accept the presence of abnormal blood flows as proof of recurrence and choose treatments accordingly without further biopsies. Most patients use the amount of decrease in number of the visible blood vessels to represent the degree of success.

MRI Complements Doppler Imaging of the Prostate

There are several MRI formats for examining the prostate. Each has its own characteristics and can refine the diagnosis. MRI routinely refers to the image of signal intensity in the gland with the patient in the tube of the unit. Three primary MRI formats have proven useful for prostate examination: EC-MRI uses an endorectal coil (EC) to improve resolution in the prostate; S-MRI or spectroscopic MRI involves analysis of the chemical composition of the prostate tissues, with emphasis on the compound *choline*; DCE (Dynamic Contrast Enhanced)-MRI is the most useful format to complement 3-D Doppler for a complete diagnosis. DCE-MRI uses the injection of a contrast agent *gadolinium* that reveals the blood flow within tumorous prostatic tissue.[4]

MRI shows cancer as a loss or decrease of the normal glandular prostatic tissue signal, however, other benign pathologies, such as calculi, hemorrhage (bleeding from recent biopsy), stones, BPH and inflammation, may also produce this effect. Some infiltrating types of cancer will not produce any visible changes. The data from the 2009 American Roentgen Ray Meeting shows a 75% sensitivity (25% false negatives) and 95% specificity (5% false positives). MRI was originally used to stage the spread of cancer outside the prostate gland also denoted as ECE (extra capsular extension). The data showed ECE medium specificity (74%) and sensitivity (71%).

Each MRI format has a unique purpose:

EC-MRI: By using the endorectal coil inflated as a balloon, EC-MRI was designed to better define the capsule of the gland and the seminal vesicles.

S-MRI: This format was designed to detect intraglandular cancer and shows the aggression. The spectroscopic chemical analysis of cancer shows higher levels of choline and citrate than in normal prostatic tissues. The analyzed sections of the prostate are divided into a grid pattern of such a size that small cancers could be missed. While this technique appeared useful for larger tumors, a 2010 *RADIOLOGY* article noted an overall sensitivity of 56% for tumor detection. Currently S-MRI is practiced at few medical centers in the US and is losing popularity at many international academic facilities. A 2008 presentation by Dr. O. Rouviere from Lyon, France at the French Radiology Meeting highlighted the problem that S-MRI was not effective in analyzing tumor extension into the fatty tissues adjacent to the prostate gland.

DCE-MRI: This format is widely used and has improved specificity by about 80% according to the 2008 *RADIOLOGY* article by Drs. J. Futterer and J. Barentsz and sponsored by the Dutch Cancer Society. DCE-MRI provides noninvasive analysis of prostate vascularization as well as tumor angiogenesis and capillary permeability characteristics in prostate cancers. (This group has also developed a 3-D S-MRI system that improves the overall accuracy of standard S-MRI.)

A fourth MRI type takes a different approach:

DWI-MRI is a process that shows molecular motion inside a tumor. The more motion, the more likely a lesion is benign, as in a fluid filled cyst. Several articles now assert that this technology may be used to predict Gleason scores. As protocols have improved, this technology is gaining wider use and clinical acceptance.

Comparing Doppler and MRI: An MRI exam shows the extent of cancer but not the activity. In patients successfully treated by radiation or hormones, the abnormality may still persist on the MRI picture; whereas, the Doppler test has the advantage of showing the blood flows are greatly reduced or completely absent. Spectroscopic MRI, (widely known as S-MRI) is also designed to show activity, but has not been shown to be as sensitive as physicians had hoped. Diffusion MRI has not been successful in finding small lesions and the EC study distorts the anatomy by the balloon inflation process. Most MRI fails to show small areas of extracapsular disease. Fortunately, the latest generation of 3D 18 mHz ultrasound probes have a resolution 5 times greater than the MRI and can verify capsule integrity. MRI is used to find spread of the prostate tumor into the boney structures, seminal vesicles and lymph nodes. It may also confirm extension of malignancy into the rectum.

Working With 3-D Doppler Imaging

The ultrasonographic physician or specially trained imaging technician looks at the instantaneous video appearing on the screen, taking pictures and measuring images according to a standard protocol, and notes and documents abnormalities. Two dimensional pictures are taken in "real time" which are similar to the images of the inside the pregnant mother's womb showing moving babies or the fetal heart beating. The same 3-D—three dimensional—technology that shows the face of the baby in the womb is now being successfully applied to the prostate. 3-D is different, in that it is faster, yet contains more information than the standard 2-D sonogram.

3-D Data Analysis: Essentially, the 3-D machine takes a volume of pictures and stores this data inside the unit's computer banks. The data may be analyzed immediately or later reviewed and reconstructed in various angles or planes. In comparing 2-D with 3-D imaging, one can say the sonographer looks and then takes pictures with the 2-D system; whereas, with the 3-D technology pictures are taken which are then looked at and formally evaluated later. If a significant problem is seen and annotated with the 2-D exam, it cannot be later observed except by completely re-scanning the patient. The 3-D rendition may be reviewed over and over without recalling and re-examining the patient. 3-D imaging has made exam time shorter providing more patient comfort. The images are then analyzed on a special computer work station allowing optimal rendering of the prostate in multiple planes as required.

Seeing Invasive Cancer: This special view, available only on 3-D equipment, allows one to see invasion of cancer more easily. Specifically, the spread of cancer outside the prostate gland or extracapsular extension is well seen with this technique.

This is critical clinical information since a tumor outside the capsule changes the cancer from operable to inoperable, and has other implications for treatment.

Individualized Assessment and Follow-Up: The patient's own vascular pattern that determines aggression can be overlaid on the 3-D scan. This adds greatly to the assessment of the disease and the feasibility of treatment possibilities unique to each individual. This is notably useful in men with low grade cancers who wish to be followed with watchful waiting, with or without nutritional or alternative therapies, thereby avoiding surgery or radiation. Most low grade tumors remain localized and may be watched or controlled with non invasive or minimally invasive treatments. (The standard MRI cannot demonstrate tumor aggression in the moment, although comparison from previous exams show progress and interval changes. 3D PDS can be repeated as often as need to objectively follow an individual.) The 3D PDS information also sets a basis for ongoing evaluation, with follow-on imaging appropriate for each individual, depending upon aggression and expectations of change, and the ability to repeat exams as often as necessary to adjust treatment based on real-time results.

2-D Standard sonogram vs. 3-D Doppler: The regular 2-D sonogram may miss low grade cancers that have the same appearance as the normal gland, which account for up to 40% of prostate tumors according to Dr. D. Downey, in the 1997 journal *UROLOGY.* The overall accuracy is about 50 %. The accuracy is better in glands that have never been subjected to a biopsy or treated in any way. The accuracy is lower in prostates that have been biopsied multiple times or in persons who have been treated with radiation or hormones.

Power Doppler: The power Doppler study adds about 30 % more accuracy, since the abnormal blood vessels provide a road map to the tumor, however, detours on the road may occur with older 3-D systems in the presence of stones or calculi. Indeed, a US patent, number 5,860,929, was obtained by Norwegian scientists to determine power Doppler blood flows in optimally diagnosing prostate cancers. When a stone is identifiable, the sound waves bounce back so strongly that they create a false color pattern. This pattern to the trained clinician will not be mistaken for a tumor vessel.

Uniquely 3-D Power Doppler Formats: Fortunately, the Doppler technology has other formats that correctly identify the artifactual or spurious colors, distinguishing it from a true cancer. In Dr. Bard's practice combining 3D PDS with focused computer aided vascular MRI exams, we have achieved a 97% overall accuracy in diagnosing and staging prostate cancers. An important exception occurs in the seminal vesicles, which sit on top of the prostate gland generating the fluid that produces the ejaculation. Early cancer spread to these paired vesicles may be missed by the 3D PDS. When a tumor is found near or adjacent to the seminal vesicles at the base of the prostate, MRI scans are mandatory. Another important advantage of 3D PDS is the ability to accurately measure tumor volume and density.

3D PDS and Tumor Volume: A meaningful use of 3-D technology is the determination of tumor volumes. Clinically "insignificant prostate cancer" is generally defined as:

1) A volume less than 0.5 cc which means the cancer is less than 7x8 mm.
2) Gleason score must be less than or equal to 7.
3) No extra-capsular extension implying: no tumor beyond the prostate capsule; no invasion of seminal vesicles; no boney metastases; and, no lymphadenopathy[1]

3D PDS and Tumor Density: Tumor density is an important factor in determining both the grade of the tumor and response to treatment. As explained elsewhere, some tumors may remain the same size or actually increase in volume while responding to treatment. Density, accurately measured by recent software advances in 3D PDS is a principal indicator of both grading, especially aggressiveness, and response to treatment on a real-time basis. (The system with this capability is FDA approved.)

The Future Potential for MRI and 3-D Doppler Ultrasound

When you look around the world at advances and innovation in MRI and 3-D Doppler technology, software and utilization, it is evident that this technology will become an important part of cancer practice, especially in this age of cost containment. Some of these techniques are not new, and are in practice outside the US. Here are just two very promising examples:

3-D Doppler: In 1999 at the University of California San Diego campus, a French medical student, Dr. Olivier Lucidarme developed a highly sensitive technique to improve Doppler ultrasound. Special bubbles injected intravenously greatly improved imaging of small vessels. To date, our FDA has not approved this technology and Dr. Lucidarme now practices this methodology in Paris at the Pitie-Salpetriere Hopital, the largest teaching center in Europe. Italian researchers at the University of Rome, Drs. Vito Cantisani and

Francesco Drudi, have shown this technology to show cancers unsuspected by other means.

MRI: Advanced MRI scans performed in Europe are not available in the US, nor are certain sophisticated radioactive bone scans, or techniques for evaluating lymph node involvement, allowed in the States at this writing. For example:

In 2004, Dr. Jelle Barentsz described a new technique to evaluate cancer spreading to the lymph nodes at the International Congress of Radiology. This uses MRI with ferumoxtran-10, a novel contrast agent called 'Combidex' in the United States. The lymph node technique is termed MRL (Magnetic Resonance Lymphangiography) and ferumaxtran-10 is being used in a wide range of MRI procedures throughout Europe, as it has shown a very good safety record, especially as it does not induce nephrogenic systemic fibrosis (NSF), a recently recognized severe complication associated with Gadolinium (Gd) based contrast agents (GBCAs) when used with patients who have compromised kidney function. GBCA is standardly used in the United States.

This technology is extremely important since MRI is the best way to image abnormal glands that are hidden or inaccessible at surgery. The imaging shows the size and location of the lymph nodes as well as the presence of cancerous tissue as small as 1/5 inch. This critical piece of information that pinpoints cancer infiltration tells where the spread occurs and allows for accurate treatment planning. The current "gold standard" for lymph node evaluation is surgery called *pelvic lymph node dissection.* Clearly this invasive exploratory operation, where the surgeon searches with his hand for hard lumps in the abdomen, cannot find all the tiny disease sites to which cancer spreads. Moreover, the metastases to nodes are generally subcentimeter so they are likely to be missed clinically and radiographically. In addition, the most reliable sign of metastatic adenopathy is in the perirectal space which is not routinely examined at surgical dissection due to its inaccessible location and surgical difficulty. The MRL exam is so accurate that a negative exam translates into a 96% chance that there is no metastatic disease to the lymph nodes. In addition to sparing patients from the risk and pain of surgery, this methodology reduces health care costs.

ProActive Monitoring — A Model
Made Possible by 3-D Doppler Technology

The monitoring approach presented here is based on Dr. Bard's thirty-nine years experience in the field of diagnostic ultrasound, fifteen years of imaging the prostate with power Doppler blood flows and six years of performing 3-D power Doppler sonograms (3D PDS) and comparing the results with high resolution MRI scans of the pelvis with special sequences formulated specifically for the prostate. Dr. Bard has diagnosed, observed and shared in the treatment of some 5,900 patients. Through nutritional support, medical treatment when appropriate, and 3-D monitoring on a schedule dictated by each individual's current situation, only five of these 5,900 men have died from their prostate cancer in a ten year time period. (This compares very favorably to the expected 239 deaths from PCa within 4 years of diagnosis, based on figures from the Health Professionals Follow-Up Study for men diagnosed with nonmetastatic PCa observed from 1990 to 2008.[6])

ProActive Monitoring couples 3-D Doppler and MRI imaging at regular intervals, with the Beta-Sitosterol/Antioxidant Matrix (B-Sit/AOX) nutritional support. The B-Sit/AOX approach was first developed out of Arthur Bartunek's early work with Co-Enzyme Q10 and cofactors that improved Q10 outcomes, especially for cancers. The formulations and protocols used during ProActive Monitoring were further refined with feedback from the progressive 3-D Doppler monitoring of men with varying stages of prostate cancer. During the 10 years of this process, improvements in imaging have allowed changes to be tracked more accurately, and to make appropriate nutritional adjustments based on this. In addition, the use of several nutritional items, notably Curcumin and Tocotrienols, have been independently developed for use with cancer and are reaching phase II and phase III clinical trials. These have been included in the protocol and are discussed here.

Beta-Sitosterol/Antioxidant Matrix (B-Sit/AOX) Nutritional Support

One way of phrasing the question we posed about ten years ago was: What could happen when essential nutrition for cell membrane integrity and healthy cell reproduction was returned to the diet through supplementation? This is a quintessential naturopathic nutritional intervention. This was based on more casual observations of improvement in PCa in men following a rigorous program of life style and dietary change. From another realm, it was observed that CoEnzyme Q10 was proving more efficacious for PCa for subjects who were also taking beta-Sitosterol rich foods, however, this was based primarily on change in PSA and not direct exam of the prostate.[7] After reviewing diets of populations with extremely low cancer, cardiovascular, and hypertension rates, a high-beta-Sitosterol based supplement was produced, with antioxidants derived from these same diets. The combination provides nutrition that is integral to cell membrane health and a healthy cell environment. Combining the B-Sit/AOX formulation with appropriate CoQ10, and a highly-rated multi-supplement with a high vitamin B Complex, became the basis for ProActive intervention. With this, watchful waiting became ProActive Monitoring.

The 3-D Color Power Doppler sonogram provides a means to track changes and progress in the condition of the prostate and PCa. By correlating the 3-D exam with state-of-the-art DCE-MRI grading of the cancer, Dr. Bard was able to both evaluate procedures for optimal timing of reexam, and provide feedback for modification the an individual's nutrition program, and in increasingly rare circumstances, recommendations for procedures such as HIFU (High-Intensity Focused Ultrasound). Routine feedback also gave the information needed to further develop the core protocol, based primarily on changes in prostate size, tumor size, location and density, vascularity, and capsule integrity.

Background – Prostate Nutrition: The walnut-sized prostate gland is a mucus-producing organ in males that lies just below the bladder. Growth to functional size is triggered by puberty, and continues until about age 30 when equilibrium is established between cell growth and apoptosis. Normal mid-life hormone changes, when coupled with diets that do not provide adequate nutrition for prostate cell integrity and hormone balance can trigger benign enlargement (BPH) and set the stage for other prostate conditions including prostatitis and prostate cancer. The typical hormone pattern leading to BPH is elevated Estradiol combined with elevated DHT, and typically estrogen dominance. This also sets up the circumstances for chronic prostatitis. While there is substantial evidence that BPH does not develop into cancer, the same underlying factors of cellular environment and integrity set the stage for PCa, and therefore, both can be considered nutritional in origin.

The key factors that influence the development of PCa include:

Inflammation: While only a relatively small percent of prostatitis – any form of inflammation of prostate tissue – is caused by bacterial infection, increasing evidence indicates a link to an imbalance in sex steroid hormones in all chronic prostatitis. Elevated levels of inflammatory cytokine IL-8 is a second and critical inflammation factor. IL-8 promotes stromal and epithelial cell proliferation. It is up-regulated in both BPH and PCa, and it is also implicated in angiogenesis. IL-8 has been shown to have a pervasive role in promoting tumor cell survival and proliferation for all cancers. Although BPH is not a causal factor for PCa, any form of chronic inflammation of the prostate can now be considered a risk factor for prostate cancer. (Some nutritional approaches have gone further, declaring inflammation the single "driving force" behind PCa and rely on non nutritive supplements in an attempt to address this issue. However, this does not restore underlying nutritional imbalances which can redress the inflammation, and adds an extra, mostly unnecessary layer of complexity.)

Prostate Cell Membrane Elasticity: There is substantial evidence from two sides that disruption in the cell membrane's elasticity increasing rigidity is a precursor for the development of cancer cells. It is also a factor in insulin resistance. On one side, there is evidence that suggests rigidity leads to focal adhesions and aberrant growth [cancer] by increasing tension in the cell that is normally generated by elevated Rho (GTP-Binding Protein family).[7,8] On the other, ultrasound units that can read the elasticity of cell membranes are now being shown to accurately be able to detect cancer. The primary dietary reason for alteration to a cell's elasticity and fluidity is an imbalance between Beta-Sitosterol (B-Sit) and cholesterol in the cell membrane.[9,10]

Membrane Permeability & Intra-Cellular Environment: There are many cell functions dependent upon normal cell membrane permeability. Of interest here is an alteration in the isoprenoid pathway, the alteration of the balance of calcium and magnesium with excessive entry of $Ca2+$ and the release of calcium stores, which is a critical factor in cancer metastasis, which can be triggered when this imbalance is accompanied by critically low CoEnzyme Q10 levels in the immediate intracellular fluids.

The same nutritional protocol described here, that addresses the above issues also increases PCa cell apoptosis, reduces proliferation, reduces excess estrogen production, supports/restores normal cell reproduction and differentiation, and reestablishes several mechanisms of homeostasis, especially for copper homeostasis. In other words, the B-Sit/AOX Matrix provides the nutritional substructure missing from today's food supply for the body's normal, dynamic anticancer functions, and when balanced properly accomplishes this at physiological levels.

Diet and Prostate Cancer: A great deal of research has been published attempting to isolate dietary factors for cancer in general, and for PCa specifically. At best, this has yielded a limited picture and conflicting recommendations. When you step back and examine the diets and food supplies of regions where cancer rates are low, a different picture emerges. For example, when the PCa rates for Greece (pre-2006) are compared to United States rates, based upon autopsy examination of the prostate, you find that men between 50 and 59 years old in Greece have a rate of 5.2%, vs. 30+% in the U.S. For men between 60 and 69 years old in Greece the rate is 13.8% while the U.S. rate is 65+%, or 4.7 times the Greek rate. This period was selected because at that time the Greek people still ate from a locally grown, heirloom food supply, unaltered in seed line and growing methods for hundreds of years (it has since changed to comply with EU requirements and their health profile appears to be rapidly changing). This food supply represents a healthy variant of the Mediterranean Diet.

In areas of Spain, where cancer rates are also extremely low, again the diet consists of locally grown heirloom-foods. From this region we have a measure of the phytosterol content of the diet, which shows that average consumption of total phytosterols is about 400 mg per day, of which 67% is beta-Sitosterol. From here if we move to Germany, where cancer rates are approximately those of the United States, again we find that the total phytosterol consumption is about 350 to 400 mg per day: however the beta-Sitosterol content is only in the 35-to-43% range.

One conclusion from this literature, especially when it is looked at in a broader context, is that it is not just the diet, but the nutritional composition of the food consumed in that diet, that makes a critical difference, and that B-Sit is essential for health in general, and our body's anti-cancer mechanisms in particular.

Another way to look as this is to look at the effects of high levels of dietary and circulating beta-Sitosterol. A partial list of the effects produced with high levels of B-Sit includes: normalizing cholesterol, a reduction in insulin resistance, support for normal weight control and fat metabolism, a reduction in asthma incidents, acting as an anti-inflammatory and an immune modulator, a reduction in cardiovascular disease and arteriolosclerosis, and reduced rates of lung, prostate, and other cancers.

Natural Synergism & Potentiation: One explanation for the wide ranging effects of adequate dietary B-Sit, which can be measured by blood levels, is that it acts in synergy with other substances, and also acts as a catalyst that potentiates antioxidant activity, as well as other antioxidant responses, especially for herb-based antioxidants, which in turn potentiate the efficacy of Vitamin D3.[11,12] It also is involved in a variety of processes throughout the body, from cell membrane structure, to regulation of estrogen and DHT production, elimination of excess estrogens, apoptosis, immune regulation, among others.

The Ideal Phytosterol Composition: Based upon the available literature and our clinical observations, the ideal balance of phytosterols is comprised of Beta-

Sitosterol being greater than 62%; Campesterol being less than 25%; Stigmasterol being less than 10 %; and Brassticasterol being less than 3%. The following is a brief summary of the evidence for this composition.

(Note: most phytosterol supplements contain a maximum of 43% Beta-Sitosterol. This is due to it being derived from currently available soy. The problem with using this material as a supplement is that is merely provides the same balance found in the food supplies that are associated with higher rates of cancer, cardiovascular disease, obesity, and type II Diabetes. Both population studies and clinical observation show that the balance of the sterols, from supplement and diet, is more important than the absolute amount. Therefore, higher supplemental amounts of properly balanced phytosterols are needed to offset the low beta-Sitosterol content and ratio from the food supply.)

Beta-Sitosterol (B-Sit): (at least 62%; absorption rate about 4%)
1. Reduces absorption of dietary cholesterol
2. High plasma concentrations are associated with a markedly reduced risk of coronary heart disease. (n 1242, >65 y/o) [13]
3. Increases apoptosis in cancer cells (4 to 6 times baseline).[14]
4. High levels in diet correlate with lower levels of cancer (prostate, lung, breast, colorectal, etc.)
5. Anti-inflammatory [14]
6. Current healthy Mediterranean food supplies provide phytosterols with over 65% beta-Sitosterol/sitostanol content, while geographical areas with high cancer and CV disease rate have about 43% or less b-SIT (with about the same amounts of total phytosterols, about 400 mg per day) content in their food. [15] U.S. intake is estimated at between 50 and 250 mg per day, with 43% or less b-Sit.[16]
7. Immune System modulator
8. Beta-Sitosterol, and Campesterol, also reduced alpha-tocopherol oxidation in liposomal membranes.
9. Decreases plaque formation in arteries.
10. Reduces Estradiol production & carries excess Estradiol from the gut.

Campesterol (CS): (not exceeding 20%; absorption rate about 13%)

1. Increases apoptosis in cancer cells (estimated to be about 4 to 6 times baseline).
2. <u>Increases</u> plaque formation in arteries.

Note: <u>Statin drugs increase CS concentrations in muscle tissue</u>, reducing b-SIT content, disrupting membrane balance. [17]

Stigmasterol: (not exceeding 10%; absorption rate about 4%)

1. Stigmasterol, but not B-Sit or CR, inhibited SREPB-2 processing and reduced cholesterol synthesis.
2. Stigmasterol activated the Liver X receptor [Liver X receptor alpha (LXRalpha), an oxysterol-activated nuclear hormone receptor, regulates the expression of genes involved in lipid and cholesterol homeostasis and inflammation.] This may improve glucose tolerance.[18]
3. However, Stigmasterol is a pro-oxidant and inflammatory.
4. Lowers Q10 levels (b-SIT & Campesterol do not)
5. Stigmasterol can cause damage to adrenal glands by disrupting normal cholesterol homeostasis. [b-SIT & CS do not]
6. And, Stigmasterol is a potent in vitro antagonist of the NR for bile acids FXR, critically involved in hepatoprotection from cholestasis (<u>inhibition of bile flow</u>).
7. [beta-Sitosterol does not have any inhibitory effect.]

Brassicasterol: (not exceeding **3%;** absorption rate not known) The European Union does not allow in supplements any amount greater then normally found in nature, which is a maximum of 3 %.

1. Brassicasterol can cause damage to adrenal glands by disrupting normal cholesterol homeostasis. [b-SIT & CS do not]
2. May lower Q10 levels [b-SIT & CS do not]

Note: Brassicasterol is significantly increased during the processing of Canola Oil. However, despite the problems with Brassicasterol for the human body, this is considered to be good, since the Brassicasterol helps stabilize the oil, and contributes to overall cholesterol lowering (#1 above).

Phytosterols Require Complementary Antioxidants

Two of the overlooked aspects of increasing dietary B-Sit is that it both stimulates the sphingomyelin cycle through increased ROS activity, increasing proliferation as demonstrated in prostate cancer cells; and high levels of both cholesterol and B-Sit can cause lipid peroxidation. For these reasons, B-Sit needs to always be administered in a composition that includes complementary antioxidants, countering the ROS activity and supporting its action in the cell membrane and intracellular environment. Regarding the effects on cancer, the practical effects of inadequate or incompatible antioxidants with B-Sit would be a leveling off at a balance between increased apoptosis and increased proliferation.

The B-Sit/AOX Matrix

The ß-Sit/AOX Matrix interaction is complex, requiring multi-supplement support. In some ways the relationship is as symbiotic as it is synergistic. For example: ß-Sitosterol potentiates antioxidant activity and activates other antioxidant responses. ß-Sit and plant-based antioxidants work together to protect cell membranes from lipid peroxidation.[19,20,21] In addition, targeted antioxidants support activities of ß-Sit: i.e. Astragalus root and ß-Sit work together to increase the activities of antioxidant enzymes, including SOD and GSH-Px[21,22].

A natural pairing of ß-Sit and select antioxidants, forming a supportive nutritional matrix, is fundamental to a wide range of biological processes, so the components of the matrix need to be selected to fit the desired outcome. In this case, the Matrix is comprised of B-Sit and antioxidants that work with it to improve membrane integrity and function, reestablish a healthy intracellular fluid environment, as well as support healthy cell reproduction and the body's mechanisms for controlling improperly reproduced cells – cancer cells.

A select group of antioxidants that form the B-Sit/AOX Matrix for natural anti-cancer support are: Astragalus, Ellagic Acid, Gynostemma Pentaphylum, Ligustrum fruit, Lutein, Lycopene, Quercetin, Resveratrol, Rhiodola, Rosemary officinalis, Schansandra fruit, trans-e-Viniferin, Wasabia japonica, and Zinc.

Synergy Within the Matrix

Just like the components that make up foods, to be efficient the Matrix needs to be comprised of nutrients that work together, for example:

- Quercetin + Resveratrol work together to naturally reduce iNOS gene expression and nitric oxide production, providing cardiovascular support and other benefits.[23]
- Resveratrol + Ellagic Acid aid the cell's structural ability to repair efficiently.[24]
- Ellagic Acid + Quercetin synergistically support normal reproduction rates and proper apoptosis when balanced at dietary-level concentrations.[25,26]
- B-Sit + Resveratrol combine to provide a balanced ROS 1 level, and synergistically inhibit inappropriate cell growth. In addition, the systemic presence of B-Sit enhances Resveratrol activity.[27]

Curcumin and B-Sit/AOX Matrix Synergy

There is growing investigation into the use of Curcumin for treatment of cancer. One of the drawbacks is the diminished effect of curcumin with increased levels of insulin. At the same time, an increased level of insulin and insulin resistance are known risk factors for developing prostate and breast cancer, as well as other cancers, and is often a cofactor with cancer patients. B-Sit reduces insulin resistance, most likely by restoring membrane function, especially selective permeability, and regulates insulin production through several mechanisms, one of which is by supporting normal cholesterol homeostasis. In addition, curcumin inhibits cell membrane cholesterol accumulation, furthering the effects of B-Sit, via a different mechanism. An ideal curcumin will be naturally absorbed, maintain effective serum levels for at least 12 hours, allowing for 24 hour effective blood levels without frequent dosing, and store in the liver for release throughout the day. In this way, doses of as little as 1,000 mg to 4,000 mg are recommended.

CoEnzyme Q10 and the B-Sit/AOX Matrix

There are a number of key reasons why CoQ10 should always be included in the Matrix. First, it is essential for proper cell reproduction. Second, it has been shown that when the circumstances for metastases are set up, the process is not triggered if there is adequate CoQ10 present. CoQ10 has been demonstrated to reduce IL-8 to normal levels. As noted above, IL-8 is the primary inflationary mechanism that drives the formation and survival of tumor cells for all cancers. Reducing IL-8 also works with the other components of the Matrix to reduce angiogenesis. The efficiency of CoQ10's function in the cell membrane and for overall cell function is restored in cancer cells through the reestablishment of membrane elasticity and permeability by B-Sit.

An ideal CoQ10 is highly absorbable and 100 % of what is supplemented needs to be available for absorption. The circulating Q10 needs to be readily able to cycle from the ubiquinone to ubiquinol forms, and be orthomolecular in nature, allowing it to be cellularly-bioavailable. Preferably, the Q10 used should have a long clinical track record and have research demonstrated efficacy. Recommended dose range is from 300 to 800 mg per day.

The above forms the basis for the nutritional support we use. As appropriate for each individual, a more complete program is developed including: Vitamin D3 to bring the D3 levels to a range of 65-to-90 ng/ml; mixed tocopherols with high gamma-tocopherol (taken in the morning) and 125 to 500 mgs of a high-delta-tocotrienol supplement taken in the evening; a balanced calcium and magnesium supplement; Vitamin K2; Vitamin B Complex; and, 5 grams of Vitamin C.

Using B-Sit/AOX Matrix Nutrition

Given that the basis of the Matrix is to restore essential missing nutrients, it can be used in a general nutrition program, during treatment, and for anyone who has developed cancer as life-long maintenance nutrition.

Monitoring & Follow-Up

The nutritional program outlined above, the **B-Sit/AOX Matrix**, has been used for over 5 years, and the results reported in the first section are based on this use. Visually, this can be seen in the following imaging of the same prostate, initially diagnosed as a Gleason 7 (Image a.) and upon a follow-up examine after daily use of the above supplement regime.

The results shown here illustrate both the efficacy of restoring fundamental nutritional support that has been systematically removed from our diets by alterations in the food supply, and the need for a means to monitor, on a regular basis, each individual's response to treatment. Given the number of factors involved in nutritional support, this is the only way to know that this individual's body is capable of restoring its anti-cancer functions. The same monitoring approach can be applied to any therapeutic intervention, especially since the 3-D sonogram is not compromised by the treatment itself.

When establishing a monitoring schedule for an individual, two additional areas need to be kept in mind, interval cancers and evaluating successful treatment.

Interval Cancers

The concept of fast growing cancers called "interval cancers" has led to routine biannual screening of male and female high risk patients. It is recognized that mammography misses invasive breast cancers with great frequency, so there is a half year time period in which health conscious women should alert themselves to the possibility of early breast cancer as they routinely undergo ultrasound breast screening twice a year. In practice, about 5 % of men develop aggressive interval cancers within half a year from their last normal or stable evaluation. A presentation *INTERVAL CANCERS OF THE PROSTATE: EVALUATION BY 3-T MRI AND 3-D POWER DOPPLER ULTRASOUND* was made at the 2011 meeting of the Societe Francaises de Radiologie in Paris demonstrating that new aggressive tumors may occur more rapidly than clinically expected and may, in part, explain the failure of certain treatments.

When a man has not had a biopsy or has had a negative biopsy and a vascular tumor is demonstrated on the 3D PDS, an MRI exam is recommended, which shows the prostate gland, the capsule of the prostate, the regional lymph glands, seminal vesicles and boney pelvis. Other bones, to which cancer frequently spreads such as the lower spine and hip, may also be imaged for abnormalities. While the MRI exam is not as good an indicator of cancer aggression, it shows spread of the tumor outside the prostate capsule to the lymph nodes better then the 3D PDS and better than the CT scan, which is currently used as the standard test for staging.

Assessing Response To Prostate Cancer Therapy

The value of medical imaging is to

- Localize volume of disease including extracapsular extension
- Assess bone metastases, seminal vesicle invasion and lymphadenopathy
- Estimate degree of aggressivity (similar to Gleason grading)
- Determine efficacy of therapy
- Monitor changes
- Tailor future therapy
- Determine tumor recurrence
- Identify new tumor

One of the problems of evaluating cancer treatment is that the tumor may be rendered harmless or even dead but the volume of the tumor remains the same or even enlarges. That is, the cancer cells may be killed off and scar tissue replaces the dead cells, leaving the size of the original malignancy unchanged or edema and necrotic fluid buildup enlarge the region simulating tumor growth. This lesson was learned 19 years ago in treating liver tumors. The therapy would render the cancer harmless, but the size of the mass on the isotope scans, sonogram, CT and MRI would remain unchanged or even enlarge. The same is true of some prostate cancers that are inactivated but still feel like cancer on the digital rectal exam and show a mass effect on the sonogram and MRI. There needs to be a way to monitor changes and determine the efficacy of treatment. Fortunately, the blood flows in malignancies that have been inactivated decrease or disappear and can be quickly and accurately measured in the moment. Thus, with 3D PDS there is a simple tool to quantify blood flow patterns to demonstrate therapeutic response.

References:

1. Ewing J. Neoplastic Diseases. 1940, WB Saunders London

2. Lassau N, Koscielny S, Avril M, Margulis A, Duvillard P, Baere T, Roche A, Leclere J. Prognostic value of angiogenesis evaluated with high frequency and color Doppler sonography for preoperative assessment of melanomas. AJR 2002;178;1547-1551

3. Cornud F, Hamida K, Flam T, Helenon O, Chretien Y, Thiounn N, Correas J, Casanova J, Moreau J. Endorectal color Doppler sonography and endorectal MR imaging features of non palpable prostate cancer. AJR 2000;175;1161-1168

4. Bard R. 2009, Dynamic Contrast Enhanced MRI of Prostate Cancer. Springer New York

5. Kenfield SA, Stampfer MJ, Giovannucci E, Chan JM. Physical Activity and Survival After Prostate Cancer Diagnosis in the Health Professionals Follow-Up Study. J Clinical Oncology. 2011 Jan 4. [Epub ahead of print]

6. Personal communication, Dr. William V. Judy and Arthur Bartunek.

7. Alexander NR, Branch KM, Parekh A, Clark ES, Iwueke IC, Guelcher SA, Weaver AM. Extracellular matrix rigidity promotes invadopodia activity. Curr Biol. 2008 Sep 9;18(17):1295-9. Epub 2008 Aug 21.

8. Choi C. Tumor malignancy linked to rigidity. The Scientist 2005, 6(1):20050919-02

9. Endress, E., S. Bayerl, K. Prechtel, C. Maier, R. Merkel, and T. M. Bayerl. The effect of cholesterol, lanosterol, and ergosterol on lecithin bilayer

mechanical properties at molecular and microscopic dimensions: A solid-state NMR and micropipet study. 2002. Langmuir 18:3293-3299.

10. Henriksen, J., A. C. Rowat, and J. H. Ipsen. 2004.Vesicle fluctuation analysis of the effects of sterols on membrane bending rigidity.Eur. Biophys. J. 33:732-741.

11. Vivancos M, Moreno JJ. b-Sitosterol modulates antioxidant enzyme response in RAW 264.7 macrophages. Free Radic Biol Med. 2005 Jul 1;39(1):91-7.

12. Wang Q, Salman H, Danilenko M, Studzinski GP. Cooperation between antioxidants and 1,25-dihydroxyvitamin D3 in induction of leukemia HL60 cell differentiation through the JNK/AP-1/Egr-1 pathway.J Cell Physiol. 2005 Sep;204(3):964-74.

13. Escurriol V, Cofan M, Moreno-Iribas C, Larranaga N, Martinez C, Navarro C, Rodriguez L, Gonzalez CA, Corella D, Ros E. Phytosterol plasma concentrations and coronary heart disease in the prospective Spanish EPIC cohort. J Lipid Res. 2009 Sep 28. [Epub ahead of print]

14. Awad AB, Fink CS. Phytosterols as Anticancer Dietary Compounds: Evidence and Mechanism of Action. J Nutr. 2000 Sep;130(9):2127-30

15. Jiménez-Escrig A, Santos-Hidalgo AB, Saura-Calixto F. Common sources and estimated intake of plant sterols in the Spanish diet. J Agric Food Chem. 2006 May 3;54(9):3462-71.

16. Cognis newsletter, October 2010

17. Päivä H, et al. High-dose statins and skeletal muscle metabolism in humans: a randomized, controlled trial. Clin Pharmacol Ther. 2005 Jul;78(1):60-8.

18. Laffitte BA, Chao LC, Li J, Walczak R, Hummasti S, Joseph SB, Castrillo A, Wilpitz DC, Mangelsdorf DJ, Collins JL, Saez E, Tontonoz P. Activation of liver X receptor improves glucose tolerance through coordinate regulation of glucose metabolism in liver and adipose tissue. Proc Natl Acad Sci U S A. 2003 Apr 29;100(9):5419-24. Epub 2003 Apr 15.

19. Moraa-Ranjeva, MP, Charveron M, Fabre B, Milon A, Muller I. Incorporation of phytosterols in human keratinocytes Consequences on UVA-induced lipid peroxidation and calcium ionophore-induced prostaglandin release. Chemistry and Physics of Lipids 2006 Jun;141(1-2):216-24.

20. Hernandez OM, Discher DJ, Bishopric NH, Webster KA. Rapid activation of neutral sphingomyelinase by hypoxia-reoxygenation of cardiac myocytes. Circ Res. 2000 Feb 4;86(2):198-204

21. Toda S, Shirataki Y. Inhibitory effects of Astragali Radix, a crude drug in Oriental medicines, on lipid peroxidation and protein oxidative modification by copper. J Ethnopharmacol. 1999 Dec 15;68(1-3):331-3.

22. Wang D, Shen W, Tian Y, Sun Z, Jiang C, Yuan S. [Protective effect of active components extracted from radix Astragali on human erythrocyte membrane damages caused by reactive oxygen species] [Article in Chinese] Zhongguo Zhong Yao Za Zhi. 1996 Dec;21(12):746-8, 763.

23. Chan MM, Mattiacci JA, Hwang HS, Shah A, Fong D. Synergy between ethanol and grape polyphenols, quercetin, and resveratrol, in the inhibition of the inducible nitric oxide synthase pathway. Biochem Pharmacol, 2000 Nov 15;60(10):1539-48.

24. Chakraborty S, Roy M, Bhattacharya RK. J. Prevention and repair of DNA damage by selected phytochemicals as measured by single cell gel electrophoresis. Enbiron Pathol Toxicol Oncol, 2004;23(3):215-26.

25. Mertens-Talcott SU, Bomser JA, Romero C, Talcott ST, Percival SS. Ellagic Acid Potentiates the Effect of Quercetin on p21waf1/cip1,p53, and MAPKinases without Affecting Intracellular Generation of Reactive Oxygen Species In Vitro. J Nutr 2005 135:609-614.

26. Mertens-Talcott SU, Talcott ST, Percival SS. Low Concentrations of Quercetin and Ellagic Acid Synergistically Influence Proliferation, Cytotoxicity and Apoptosis in MOLT-4 Human Lukemia Cells. J Nutr 2003 133:2669-2674.

27. Vivancos M, Moreno JJ, Effect of resveratrol, tyrosol and ß-sitosterol on oxidised low-density lipoprotein-stimulated oxidative stress, arachidonic acid release and prostaglandin E2 synthesis by RAW 264.7 macrophages. British J of Nutr 2008 99:1199-1207

INSPIRATION: ONE WOMAN'S JOURNEY WITH BREAST CANCER

My Story

Donna Ranaudo Kraus

On July 25th 1999, I examined my breasts for the first time and found a lump in my left breast. It was the size of an olive and was as hard as a rock.

Two days later I was diagnosed with stage 1 breast cancer.

Three days later I had surgery, a partial mastectomy. Thankfully, it was only in my breast and it didn't spread anywhere else. I was very lucky. Medullary carcinoma of the breast is a less common form of invasive breast cancer. It is found in only 3 to 5% of all breast cancers diagnosed.

At the time I was living a very healthy lifestyle; I ate a vegan diet, took my supplements and, for the most part, treated myself holistically. I had always known that if a serious illness ever struck me, like cancer, I would treat it holistically. What I wasn't prepared for when I heard the word "cancer," was the paralyzing fear I felt. It gripped me so tightly that it made me second guess everything I ever believed in.

After the surgery, I was faced with choosing a path to prevent a recurrence. My breast surgeon, Dr. Cahan, recommended radiation. To my surprise, I seriously considered it and began to open my mind to the possibility of chemo and radiation. My only thought was to make sure the cancer was truly gone, and that it would never come back.

I made appointments with three highly respected oncologists to determine my next course of action. The first doctor told me to do chemo, the second doctor recommended radiation, and the third doctor said the best choice was to do both.

They each said their opinion would provide the best chance at my ultimate health. The problem was, they weren't in agreement with each other. These three prominent doctors each gave their educated opinions, in great detail with statistical evidence, but each opinion was different.

Who was I to believe? Who was right, and more importantly, how was I supposed to choose? This is my life we're talking about. How do I figure out who to trust with my life? These relentless thoughts sent me into a tailspin and I began to have debilitating panic attacks. I was terrified, angry, sad and totally confused. Still, I kept my focus—I was determined to figure this whole thing out. Ultimately, I had no other choice but to take matters into my own hands.

During this time I received a phone call from a woman who belonged to Reach to Recovery. This organization was affiliated with the hospital, and called patients after surgery to check on them and make sure they are recovering properly. After a two hour uplifting conversation, this woman told me about a complementary medicine cancer support group at Benedictine Hospital and a woman named Hope Nemiroff, who helped run it.

Hope had been a survivor for over 5 years. I went to visit her and learn her survival story. She welcomed me into her home and we spent over four hours talking. She gave me detailed information on what she did and what she learned along her journey. Hope gave me books, reputable websites, audio tapes, VHS tapes, transcripts and a list of doctors that used both conventional therapies and alternative therapies.

What I valued the most was the way Hope NEVER told me what to do and never said she had all the answers. She just urged me to inform myself so that I could make an educated decision about what I was going to do next—and I did. I went on a three month crusade, researching both conventional and alternative therapies and interviewing everyone who had survived cancer.

After my third month of intense research, I came to a decision. I chose not to do chemo or radiation and to go the alternative route. It was the most difficult choice to make since I was going against the norm, but it was a well-informed, well educated decision. I knew in my heart it was the right choice for me.

In November of 1999, I made my first appointment with Dr. Schachter (see below) and I have never looked back. In September of 2000, I started working at the health food store Nature's Pantry, (www.naturespantryny.com). To this day, on a regular basis, customers battling cancer ask me what I did to beat this disease. I tell each of them how I educated myself and how I had a full understanding of all the options before I chose the all natural path. Ultimately I did what I felt was best for ME.

Here is my advice to you - Research and fully understand all of your options completely, and then go with your GUT. Do what feels right inside for you, and don't let anyone talk you into doing what *they* think is best. Knowledge is power; the more you know, the better the choices you will make and the more confident you will be in that choice.

I decided to write my story and share it, just like Hope did for me. The following is my personal journey; my doctors, books, websites, support groups, supplements, mind/body medicine and other information I have learned along the way that has been successful in both preventing and treating cancer.

My Personal Doctors
Dr. Michael Schachter M.D.
845-368-4700
www.mbschachter.com
Schachter Center for Complimentary Medicine
2 Executive Blvd
Suffern, NY 10901

I have been under Dr. Schachter's care since November 1999 to prevent a recurrence of breast cancer. He is a medical doctor who uses an alternative approach to treat cancer and other diseases. His objective is to get to the underlying cause of the disease so he can effectively treat that and the symptoms. He taps into the body's natural ability to heal itself by building up the immune system, and blending both conventional and alternative medicine to achieve optimal health. An individualized holistic treatment plan is developed for each patient.

He is featured in Chapter 18 of the book "Alternative Medicine: The Definitive Guide to Cancer." He is also referenced in Suzanne Somer's book "Knockout". I have seen miraculous things happen at Dr. Schachter's office. Patients shared their stories with me who were sent home with only six months to live, and under Dr. Schachter's treatment they beat the odds by surviving 3, 5, and even 9 years past their death sentences.

Dr. Anthony Cahan M.D.

914-517-8263

www.nwhc.net

The Breast Institute at NWH

6400 East Main Street

Mt Kisco, NY 10549

White Plains Office 914-681-9481

Dr. Cahan is my breast surgeon. He is currently the Chief of Breast Surgical Services at Northern Westchester Hospital in Mount Kisco. When I made my decision to go alternative, I discussed this with Dr. Cahan. He was honest and told me he wasn't in agreement with me and he urged me to do radiation. I told him I respected his opinion and asked him if he would respect mine, and still continue to be my doctor. He said he would; He'd rather have me as a patient than to see me leave without any follow up examinations. I am very grateful to him. Most doctors would not have done that, and I would have been on my own. I continue to see him every six months and will do so for the rest of my life.

Dr. Robert Bard M.D.

212-355-7017

www.cancerscan.com

121 East 60th Street,

New York, NY

Dr. Bard is my radiologist. He specializes in power Doppler sonography, which can detect a malignancy when it is 1/4 inch in size. It is highly accurate, especially in high risk patients with lumpy breasts (where mammograms are of limited diagnostic value). Power Doppler sonography is a simple test that shows the blood flow in abnormal vessels. The combined use of breast sonograms with Doppler blood flow study will provide early detection of most highly malignant cancers, resulting in life-saving early diagnosis and sparing patients radical surgery.

Dr. Peter Kaplan – Psychologist
www.drpeterkaplan.com
845-255-1440
62 Rocky Hill Road
New Paltz, NY 12561

Managing Stress

One of the key things to staying healthy is to learn how to manage your stress. This has been my biggest challenge throughout my journey. When I was first diagnosed with cancer, I began having severe panic attacks. I was terrified of my uncertain future. I constantly worried about dying and leaving my son motherless. I stressed over leaving my immediate family and how this would affect them. I was especially worried about my husband, who had already lost three family members to cancer and was still dealing with those tremendous losses. I couldn't get a grip and was becoming unglued, paralyzed by my negative thoughts.

I spoke to my doctor about it and he recommended that I see a therapist, Dr. Peter Kaplan. This man changed my life completely. I tell people that he literally saved me during the most difficult time of my life, and I will be forever grateful to him.

On my first visit with Dr. Kaplan, he outlined his approach and the different treatment options he uses to help people overcome anxiety.

The first plan of attack was biofeedback. Biofeedback is an interactive computer program that monitors your physical and emotional responses to stress. The machine is attached to the patient's fingertips, and provides visual feedback on the screen. It teaches you how to bring yourself out of a panic and into a balanced state through deep breathing and guided imagery. Biofeedback played an intricate part in controlling my panic attacks. I actually still use it today through a program called Healing Rhythms. This biofeedback program is available for use on your personal home computer and can be found at www.wilddivine.com.

In addition to biofeedback, Dr. Kaplan gave me the tools I needed to manage my life and daily challenges. I now have this tool box for life, and I continue to use it daily to keep me from going back to that dark place. I also utilized many books, tapes and other resources to change my negative thinking pattern while I was still in therapy (see guided imagery below). I took yoga, meditation classes and a seminar called The Journey (see below).

One of the most significant questions Dr. Kaplan asked as if I was in touch with my spiritual side. When I was diagnosed, my cousin Marie urged me to start praying and to go back to church. I hadn't been to church in several years. She was insistent and begged me to go before my surgery, so I did, even though I felt like a hypocrite. After my surgery I began to go to church every Sunday and to pray regularly. It felt good, but something was still missing and this was something we discussed in therapy. These intense sessions ultimately led me to pursue a personal relationship with God. With this renewed relationship, through prayer and studying, I found freedom from my fears, a comforting sense of peace, and an inner knowing that I am truly not alone.

Diet

Most people do not understand the power of food. It has the power to make you very sick, but it also has the healing power to cure and prevent diseases. Educating yourself on what you should eat and what you should avoid will dramatically strengthen your immune system and can ultimately help you win the battle against cancer. The following information is just a start on how you can improve your health through diet; don't try to change everything all at once, as you will set yourself up for failure. I believe that if you add something beneficial to your diet each week, and at the same time eliminate something unhealthy, you will win the diet battle.

Cancer Fighting Foods

Eat organic foods as much as possible. A diet made of whole, unprocessed foods, such as green leafy vegetables, fruit, whole grains, sprouted grains, legumes, seeds, nuts and sea vegetables helps to put the body into an alkaline environment. Fresh vegetable juices provide live enzymes that are easily absorbed and reach down to cellular levels to nourish and enhance growth of healthy cells. If you eat red meat, limit it to once a week and make sure it's organic beef. All animal products, including chicken, turkey, etc., must be organic. As a rule, your food should be steamed, baked or lightly sautéed. Drink pure, non-chlorinated and non-fluoridated water.

The following is a list of specific cancer fighting diet books:

- The Cure is in the Kitchen: The Strict Healing Phase for the Macrobiotic Diet by Sherry Rogers
- Ultimate Detox Diet by Teri Kerr

- Beating Cancer with Nutrition by Patrick Quillin
- What to Eat if you have Cancer by Maureen Keane
- The PH Miracle Diet by Robert Young & Shelly Redford Young
- The Self-Healing Cookbook by Kristina Turner
- Eat Right 4 Your Blood Type by Dr. Peter D'Adamo

If you need help with restructuring your diet, I recommend seeing a nutritionist in your area to work with you one-on-one directly. If you decide to see Dr. Schachter, he has a nutritionist on staff that can help you. If you live in the Hudson Valley, I recommend Sarah LaVallee. Sarah specializes in helping others achieve their health goals through proper nutrition, supplementation, and wellness exercises. For more information please visit her website at www.yournaturalbody.com.

Avoid List

Sugar – Avoid foods containing added sugars (cakes, cookies, candies, ice cream, sodas, sugar cereals, condiments, etc.)

Acceptable: Sugar natural to food, such as the sugar in fruit, raw unfiltered honey, unsulphured black strap molasses, pure maple syrup, rice syrup, date sugar, agave nectar, and stevia. Use these in moderation.

Alcohol – Avoid all alcoholic beverages, including liquor, beer and wine. Try naturally sparkling spring water with a twist of lemon or lime as your social drink.

Caffeine – Avoid coffee, tea, soda and chocolate as much as possible. Also avoid decaffeinated coffee, since chemicals are used in the decaffeination process. If you must drink coffee, it should be organic, because most coffee is high in pesticides. Herbal teas are acceptable substitutes, and often have therapeutic properties.

White Flour Products – Avoid white bread, white pasta products and white rice. Whole grain flour products and brown rice are a more nutritious, acceptable substitute. . However, some people have problems with wheat and gluten, or have celiac disease; and need to avoid whole grains altogether.

Hydrogenated Oil – Avoid hydrogenated fats, which are just oils that have been made hard by the addition of hydrogen atoms (margarine, Crisco, mayonnaise, and processed peanut butter, etc.). They contain trans fatty acids. Most packaged foods, like cereal and cookies, will have partially hydrogenated oil in their list of ingredients. You *must* read labels.

Acceptable oils: nut butters that are not hydrogenated, saturated fats (butter, animal fats, coconut and palm oil) are allowed in moderation. Unsaturated cold pressed vegetable oils (safflower, sesame, sunflower, virgin olive oil) may be used. Olive oil or broth may be used for sautéing.

Additives/Preservatives– Again labels MUST BE READ. Avoid artificial preservatives (BHA, BHT, MSG, nitrites, nitrates, sodium benzoate, etc.) commonly found in bread, crackers, cereals, cakes, cookies. Avoid all processed cured meats, such as bologna, salami, hot dogs, corned beef and pastrami. These nitrates produce carcinogenic nitrosamines. Avoid the artificial coloring and artificial flavoring (identified as natural flavors) commonly found in ice creams, frozen pies and candy. Avoid the bromine & bromide found in commercially baked goods. Avoid all artificial sweeteners, such as aspartame (Nutrasweet), sucralose (Splenda), and saccharine (Sweet 'n Low). All diet sodas, diabetic foods, and other processed low calorie foods should be avoided since they most likely contain artificial sweeteners. Acceptable substitutes are found in your local health food store.

Fluoride – Avoid fluoridated water and all tap water, unless filtered appropriately. Avoid fluoride-containing supplements, toothpaste and dental fluoride treatments. To filter fluoride from tap water, the filter must contain a reverse osmosis component. Toothpaste without fluoride and containing all natural ingredients may be purchased at most health food stores. Chlorinated water should be filtered to remove chlorine.

Genetically Modified Foods – All GMO's should be avoided as much as possible. Please visit www.geneticroulette.com for more information.

Tobacco – Do not smoke and try to avoid inhaling other people's smoke as much as possible.

Recreational Drugs – Avoid unnecessary prescription drugs and OTC medication. We are an over-medicated society. Medication related deaths are the fourth leading cause of death in our country.

Synthetic Hormones – These are found in hormone replacement therapy and birth control pills. If there is a need, bio-identical hormones may be used if monitored carefully.

Mercury, Amalgam/Dental fillings – Mercury is highly toxic and enters the tissues of the body to damage the nervous system and immune system. Vaccines containing thimerosal, a preservative containing mercury, are potentially dangerous and should be avoided as much as possible.

Tight clothing – Do not wear anything that can restrict lymphatic system drainage. Bras, especially those worn for more than twelve hours, may restrict this and may be associated with breast cancer.

Aluminum Cookware – Along with Teflon cookware, this should be avoided because aluminum tends to accumulate in the body and fluoride may be released from the Teflon.

Antiperspirant Deodorants – Avoid all deodorants that contain aluminum because it inhibits detoxification of the breasts and chest area.

Synthetic Hair Dyes – These dyes contain ammonia and lead and may increase your risk for cancer. Certain natural dyes sold in health food stores are acceptable.

High Voltage Power Lines – Avoid power lines as much as possible. If your home is located near them, consider moving.

Microwave

- Do not use plastic containers or plastic wrap in the microwave. The combination of high heat and plastics releases dioxins into the food, which are highly poisonous to the cells of our bodies.

- Do not put your water bottles in freezer. Freezing plastic water bottles also releases dioxins from the plastic. Instead, use glass or ceramic containers for heating food. You get the same results, only without the dioxin. So TV dinners, instant ramen and soups, etc., should be removed from the container before heating.

Supplements

The following is a list of supplements that I have learned to be successful in battling cancer. Please consult your doctor before taking. Asterisks indicate those I have personally taken.

Amygdalin – Amygdalin is also known as Vitamin B17 or Laetrile. It is a derivative of Apricot Seeds and is known to be lethal to cancer cells but not to the rest of your body. In clinical trials, Amygdalin showed the stoppage of metastases (the spread of cancer). Please read more detail about this supplement in my section on Dr. Ralph Moss.

IP6 (Inositol) – Research shows that **IP6 (Inositol)** is a potent antioxidant and boosts natural killer (NK) cell activity. More importantly, it helps to normalize the rate of cell division of uncontrolled or cancerous cells. NK cells are immune system defense cells that target not only cancerous cells, but also virally infected cells. As a result, a very wide range of immune-related conditions, from the common cold to hepatitis, may benefit from IP6.

CoQ10 – Coenzyme Q10 is used by our bodies to produce energy. It is an antioxidant that protects us from free radical damage and stimulates the immune system.

Selenium – The mineral selenium has been shown in multiple studies to be an effective tool in warding off various types of cancer. In addition to preventing the onset of the disease, selenium has also been shown to aid in slowing cancer's progression in patients that already have it.

Dr. Bard's PMCaox – This antioxidant cell protection formula was developed by Dr. Bard to naturally address the nutrition concerns of women including the promotion of healthy breast tissue, GYN health, hormone balance, cardiovascular health, free radical protection, immune support, energy and stress.

Iodine – Through the 1800's and early 1900's iodine was used extensively to cure many illnesses, including **cancer**, **goiter,** infections, thyroid, skin problems, lung conditions, and autoimmune conditions.

Fish Oil – Researchers found that a high intake of fish oil significantly lowered the cancer incidence in animal studies, compared to animals fed either low fat diets or high corn oil diets. By implanting human tumors into immune-deficient mice, researchers have found that a high fish oil diet can slow tumor growth. These results suggest that fish oil can be used for both the prevention and treatment of cancer.

FlorEssence – "Essiac" as known in the market place today is comprised of 4 herbs: Sheep Sorrel (Rumex acetosella), Burdock Root (Arctium lappa), Slippery Elm Bark (Ulmus fulva), and Turkish Rhubarb Root (Rheum palmatum). This 4-herb formula is a smaller version to the original formula by Canadian nurse Rene Caisse. "Essiac" began decades ago when Rene Caisse heard of an herbal recipe from an elderly female patient, who was in the Ontario hospital where Rene was head nurse.

The recipe contained 8 herbs, given to the woman years before by an Ojibway medicine man. He offered his help, because he knew the woman was suffering from breast cancer. The patient recovered from her cancer and saw no return during the next 30 years. In 1922, she gave Rene the recipe when Rene thought it could possibly help others.

Flaxseed – Flaxseed and its oil have been promoted since the 1950's as a dietary nutrient with anti-cancer properties. The oil extracted from flaxseeds is said to lower cholesterol levels, boost the immune system, and prevent cancer.

Vitamin A – Doctors' experience and clinical evidence both show that vitamin A helps prevent cancer. The association between vitamin A and cancer was initially reported in 1926 when rats, fed a vitamin A-deficient diet, developed gastric carcinomas.

Vitamin D – Research indicates that vitamin D, whether produced in the skin from exposure to sunlight, from sun lamps or obtained from supplementation, helps cancer patients. Proper vitamin D supplementation gives one a much better chance of preventing many major illnesses such as, cancer, heart disease, hypertension, arthritis, chronic pain, depression, inflammatory bowel disease, obesity, premenstrual syndrome, muscular weakness, fibromyalgia, crohns disease, multiple sclerosis and autoimmune illness.

Vitamin E – Antioxidants, such as vitamin E, help protect against the damaging effects of free radicals, which may contribute to the development of chronic diseases like cancer. Vitamin E may also protect against the development of cancers by enhancing immune function.

Garlic – Many studies showed that the main ingredient of garlic, allyl sulfur, is effective in inhibiting or preventing cancer development. Out of 37 studies, 28 studies showed evidence that garlic can prevent cancer. It is thought that the allyl sulfur compounds in garlic prevent cancer by slowing or preventing the growth of the cancer tumor cells.

Chinese Herbs/Acupuncture – Traditional Chinese Medicine is an ancient system of healing that bases diagnosis on an individual's pattern of symptoms, rather than looking for a named disease. **To find a knowledgeable Chinese herbologist, visit** www.acupunctureamerica.com

Milk Thistle – Laboratory studies suggest that silymarin and the other active substances in milk thistle may have anti-cancer effects. These substances appear to stop cancer cells from dividing and reproducing, shorten their life span, and reduce blood supple to tumors.

Green Tea* – Animal studies suggest that green tea increases cancer cell death and suppresses blood vessel growth in cancer.

Cat's Claw – Cat's claw (*Uncaria tomentosa*) is a plant most often imported from the rainforests of Peru. Its inner bark is used for a variety of medicinal purposes. It contains a group of alkaloids that are thought to possess anti-cancer and antitumor activity and stimulate the immune system.

Carnivora – Carnivora is the 100% pure phytonutrient extract of Dionaea Muscipula, a particular species of the Venus flytrap plant. It works very well for early stage cancers, with a good success rate for more advanced cancers. For more information visit www.carnivora.com

Moldifilan* – Moldifilan is the purest, most organic extract of the brown seaweed Laminaria Japonica. This extract contains the life essential properties of organic iodine, alginates, fucodian and laminarin. Organic iodine regulates metabolism and promotes maturation of the nervous system. Alginate is a natural absorbent of radioactive elements, heavy metals and free radicals. Fucoidan kills cancer cells. Laminarin is a polysaccharide helpful in the prevention and treatment of cardiovascular disease. Visit www.moldifilan.com to learn more.

Mushrooms

- Maitake (Grifola frondosa) is an edible mushroom. In addition to its anti-cancer, anti-viral and immune-enhancing properties, maitake may also reduce blood pressure and stabilize blood sugar.

- Reishi (Ganoderma lucidum) is too bitter to eat but is widely available in tea bags, capsules and liquid extracts. Animal studies have shown that reishi improves immune function and inhibits the growth of some malignant tumors.

- Agaricus blazei, now known as Agaricus brasiliensis, contains beta glucans, a group of polysaccharides (complex sugars) believed responsible for this mushroom's immune-boosting effects. Research has shown that Agaricus blazei has anti-tumor and anti-viral activity, as well as moderating effects on blood sugar and cholesterol. Oncologists in both Japan and Brazil use this mushroom in treatment protocols. It is sold in the U.S. in dried form as well as in extracts.

Recommended Doctors/ Wellness Practitioners

Dr. Stanislaw Burzynski M.D. www.burzynskiclinic.com 800-714-7181 9432
Burzynski Clinic
Katy Freeway, Suite 200
Houston, Texas 77055

Dr. Burzynski is not my personal doctor; he is an internationally recognized physician and scientist who has devoted his whole life to cancer research. He has been treating thousands of cancer patients from all parts of the world for over thirty years. Dr. Burzynski is known worldwide for discovering Antineoplastons, a therapy that targets cancer cells without destroying normal cells. Dr. Schachter invited me to the Gary Null PBS seminar, and I had the pleasure of meeting Dr. Burzynsky and several of his patients, who have survived more than twenty-five years. He spoke in detail about this therapy and his patients' successes. Please visit his website to learn more.

Gary Null PhD www.garynull.com
2307 Broadway
New York, NY 10024

For over three decades, Gary Null has been one of the foremost advocates of alternative medicine and natural healing. He has been a consistent voice on how to live a longer, more vital life through work that embraces the body, mind and spirit.

Gary's philosophy has influenced countless people to achieve a healthier, more fulfilling lifestyle. He is the author of over 70 books on nutrition and self empowerment. In April, 2009 Gary asked Dr. Schachter, Dr. Burzynski, and several other doctors if they would come to his headquarters in NYC to do a special for PBS about cancer patients who have survived using alternative methods. The doctors brought their patients who had successfully beaten cancer by using alternative therapies. Dr. Schachter asked me, and I was honored to go and tell my story. That was where I met Dr. Buryzinski and so many others who survived cancer and beat the odds.

Recommended Research

Healing Therapies
Dr. Ralph Moss M.D
www.ralphmoss.com/html/mossOTA.shtml The Moss Reports

Dr. Moss is not my personal doctor, but one that I researched heavily. His findings played a very big part in the choices I made during my battle against cancer. Dr. Ralph Moss is a well respected doctor who worked for Sloan Kettering. In 1975, he met with a Dr. Sugiura, a scientist who was working on the cancer killing power of Laetrile, also known as Vitamin B17 or Amygdalin(a derivative of apricot seeds).

Dr. Moss discovered that Dr. Sugiura's clinical trials on Amygdalin showed that small tumors stopped growing for a period of time and then started growing again. This was significant because it was the discovery of the stoppage of metastases.

These were the greatest results ever achieved in cancer. He was excited about this discovery, especially since he had never believed in Laetrile.

Dr. Moss found out that Sloan Kettering knew of these findings and had covered up of the results on Laetrile. So Dr. Moss blew the whistle on this cover up, and was fired the next day for failing to lie on behalf of Memorial Sloan Kettering. Please visit his website to find out his story and the amazing results of Amygdalin.

When I was first diagnosed, I chewed these seeds raw, took Amygdalin 500mg tablets, and had it administered intravenously at Dr. Schachter's. I purchase them from Mexico because it is unavailable in the U.S. The FDA will not allow it. I still take it every day for prevention. It is lethal to cancer cells, just like chemotherapy, but does not harm the rest of your body.

Jason Vale

If you go to the website www.apricotsfromgod.com, you will learn about Jason Vale. This man cured himself of cancer with apricot seeds. I had the honor of talking to Jason when I was first diagnosed, and purchased the seeds from him. He is an amazing human being.

As a result of him trying to help people with cancer and informing the public about apricot seeds, he was locked up and put in jail by the FDA. He spent five years of his life in jail just because he wanted everyone to know there was another option out there to fight this horrible disease. I am still shocked at what happened to him; he just wanted to share with people how he beat cancer, and he paid a very high price for his generosity. Please visit his website and read his story, you will be outraged.

Deepak Chopra, M.D.
www.deepakchopra.com or www.chopra.com
Mind/Body Healing

Deepak Chopra and David Simon, M.D., opened the Chopra Center for Wellbeing in 1996 to help people experience physical healing, emotional freedom, and higher states of consciousness. The center is located in Carlsbad, California, and they integrate the healing arts of the East with the best in modern Western medicine. He offers interactive courses and trainings plus books, CD's and DVD's in yoga, meditation, etc. I spent many years listening to him and am grateful for his teachings.

Dr. Wayne Dyer PH.D
www.drwaynedyer.com
Mind/Body Healing

Wayne Dyer is an internationally renowned author and speaker in the field of self-development. He is the author of over thirty books, has created many audio programs and videos, and has appeared on thousands of television and radio shows. He is called the "father of motivation" by his fans. He has overcome many obstacles to make his dreams come true. Today, he spends much of his time showing others how to do the same. Just like Deepak, I spent many years listening to Wayne, and I am grateful for his teachings, as well.

Dr. Andrew Weil M.D. www.drweil.com

Dr. Andrew Weil is a Harvard-trained medical doctor and world-renowned pioneer in integrative medicine. He developed **A Step-by-Step Plan for Mind, Body, and Spirit**. Dr. Weil has helped thousands of people achieve better health and wellness with this customized practical plan of action to help you feel your best and prevent future illness.

Suzanne Somers www.suzannesomers.com

Suzanne used an alternative approach to healing her own cancer and has written several books about it, including Breakthrough & Knockout. She is also known for her books on anti aging and her Somersize diet. You can read up on Suzanne Somers on her website.

The Journey by Brandon Bays
www.thejourney.com

The Journey is the actual life work of Brandon Bays. Brandon explains how she healed from a basketball-size tumor in 6½ weeks with no drugs or surgery. This is healing on the cellular level, from diseases like cancer and physical illnesses to issues like anxiety, depression, stress, chronic pain, anger, and low self-esteem. After I read this book, I went to her seminar in NYC. It was very powerful and completely shifted something in me. Forgiveness is extremely powerful in healing yourself and it is the heart of what "The Journey" is all about.

Suggested Reading

*What Your Doctor May Not Tell You About Breast Cancer by John Lee

*Alternative Medicine Definitive Guide to Cancer by W. John Diamond, W. Lee Cowden with Burton Goldberg

*Encyclopedia of Healing Therapies by Anne Woodham and Dr. David Peters

*Prescription of Nutritional Healing by Phyllis A. Balch

*Healthy Healing by Linda Page, PH.D

Healing Therapies

Acupuncture is one of the main forms of treatment in traditional Chinese medicine. It involves the use of sharp, thin needles that are inserted in the body at very specific points. This process is believed to adjust and alter the body's energy flow into healthier patterns, and is used to treat a wide variety of illnesses and health conditions.

Homeopathy, or homeopathic medicine, is a holistic system of treatment that originated in the late eighteenth century. The system is based on the idea that the same substances which produce symptoms of sickness in healthy people will have a curative effect when given in very dilute quantities to the sick who exhibit those same symptoms. Homeopathic remedies are believed to stimulate the body's own healing processes.

Chiropractic is one of the most popular alternative therapies currently available. It is grounded in the principal that the body can heal itself when the skeletal system is correctly aligned and the nervous system is functioning properly. To achieve this, the practitioner uses his or her hands or an adjusting tool to perform specific manipulations of the vertebrae.

Guided Imagery/Visualization is defined in the Alternative Medicine Encyclopedia as "the use of relaxation and mental visualization to improve mental and physical wellbeing." It is a two part process that uses deep breathing and imagery. Dr. Emmet Miller has wonderful CD's that will help change an unwanted behavior and insert the behavior you want to develop. This is software for the mind at its best. Several imagery experiences build confidence, re-script the past, and help create an exciting new future as negative self images and habits are replaced with positive ones. Visit www.drmiller.com for more information.

Applied Kinesiology is the study of muscles and the relationship of muscle strength to health. It incorporates a system of manual muscle testing and therapy. AK is based on the theory that an organ dysfunction is accompanied by a specific muscle weakness. Diseases are diagnosed through muscle-testing procedures and then treated.

Yoga combines physical exercises, mental <u>meditation</u> and breathing techniques to strengthen muscles, improve flexibility, alleviate physical symptoms, relieve stress and increase general health.

Meditation is a practice of concentrated focus upon a sound or object with deep breathing in order to increase awareness of the present moment. Meditating daily will reduce **stress**, promote relaxation, and enhance personal and spiritual growth.

Lymphatic Drainage is a massage of the lymph system to detoxify and reduce the risk of infection after surgery or cancer treatment. Locate a capable practitioner of lymphatic drainage massage in your area.

Colonics are also called colon hydrotherapy and colonic irrigation. A colonic cleanse is the process in which purified water is flushed through the colon via the rectum, in order to remove waste products that may become breeding grounds for illness-causing bacteria. Search the web for a colon therapist near you.

Stem Cell – There are a variety of diseases and injuries in which a patient's cells or tissues are destroyed and must be replaced by tissue or organ transplants. Stem cells may be able to generate brand new tissue in these cases, and even cure diseases for which there currently are no adequate therapies. Diseases that could see revolutionary advances using stem cell research include cancer, Alzheimer's and Parkinson's, <u>diabetes</u>, <u>spinal cord injuries</u>, <u>heart disease</u>, stroke, <u>arthritis</u> and burns.

Exercise

Cancer cells cannot thrive in an oxygenated environment. Exercising daily and deep breathing exercises help get more oxygen down to the cellular level. Oxygen therapy is another means employed to destroy cancer cells.

Support Groups/Dutchess County

Breast Cancer Options

www.breastcanceroptions.org

This is an organization born out of the original support group I joined when first diagnosed. It is run by Hope Nemiroff, the very same survivor who spent all those hours with me. BCO is an organization of survivors and their supporters, who understand that a woman diagnosed with breast cancer is suddenly faced with some of the most important decisions she will ever make about her own healthcare. In deciding on a plan of action, it is important to understand that you do not have to face all this, including physician visits, by yourself. The support group meetings have a few locations; please visit the website for the location closest to you.

Miles of Hope Breast Cancer Foundation

www.milesofhopebcf.org

This is non-profit foundation has a mission to provide funds to support programs for people affected by breast cancer in the Hudson Valley. They offer a wide range of services to support the patient and their families during such a difficult time. For more detailed information, please visit their website.

Remember, cancer is a disease of the body, mind, and spirit. A proactive and positive spirit will help the cancer warrior become a survivor. Anger, grudges, and bitterness put the body into a stressful and acidic environment. Learn to have a loving, forgiving spirit and to relax and enjoy life.

Donna Ranaudo Kraus~beachgirl1212@gmail.com~845-831-8549

CPSIA information can be obtained at www.ICGtesting.com
Printed in the USA
LVOW01s1731200214

374550LV00005B/13/P

9 781614 489054